Praise for *Well Being*

*"These days it's becoming rarer to come across a soul whose
intentions for healing and life betterment are directed to others instead
of solely directed to themselves. Not only is Valentina's focus on others and
their healing, but she also possesses a special level of compassion
that she directs into everything she does in her life's work."*

— **Anthony William**, Medical Medium, #1 *New York Times* best-selling author

*"The mere absence of disease is not health. True health occurs when we
see improvement in every domain of our well-being. Honest and engaging,
Valentina Gaylord's book explores how to approach creating true health."*

— **Shawn Achor**, *New York Times* best-selling author of
Big Potential and *The Happiness Advantage*

"In Well Being, *Valentina shares her transformational experience
to validate and illuminate the process of healing. In the midst of my own
journey to health, her book offered reassurance of being on the right path.
Thank you, Valentina, for the terrific insights and vulnerable sharing
of your journey. You have given this Olympian inspiration to push
ahead to meet my health and wellness goals!"*

— **Greg Louganis**, world-renowned diver, four-time Olympian,
and winner of four gold medals and one silver medal

*"Valentina writes an amazingly deep and vulnerable story of her own hard-
earned healing and reclaiming of a life that better serves the entirety of the
body in all its forms. I highly recommend this book for anyone who feels alone
in their struggle to find and forge their own path to whole-body healing."*

— **Emily A. Francis**, author of *The Body Heals Itself*

"In Well Being, *Valentina Gaylord not only relates her own
inspiring journey to wellness. She also helps readers chart their
own journeys in a deeply personal way. Her incisive questioning and
compassionate guidance create a framework for each of us to
write our own story of healing in body, mind, and soul."*

— **Nadia Comăneci**, first gymnastics perfect ten in Olympic history,
five-time Olympic Gold Medalist, and winner of
three silver medals and one bronze medal

"I believe Valentina to be a light and a guidepost to life.
If you would like a breather from the storms of your life and your soul,
I recommend her authentic words about her struggles and healing. I found
comfort in the way she puts forth a compassion for life and a willingness
to look where things are never comfortable. Everyone deserves
'well being,' but you have to look for it!"

— **Peter Barton**, film and television actor

"In Well Being, *Valentina Gaylord has created a resource that is
empowering and deeply moving. Her ability to articulate the nuanced
steps of healing, both physical and emotional, provides a compassionate
and practical road map for those navigating their paths to recovery and self-
discovery. Her wisdom and empathetic approach offer readers the tools
they need to overcome obstacles and foster a resilient spirit. Her words
offer solace, strength, and guidance, making this book an essential
companion for anyone committed to their healing journey."*

— **Tatiana Gutsu**, Olympic Gold Medalist, CEO
and president of Empowerment Zone and Worldwide Gift of Fit

"*Valentina Gaylord's* Well Being *is the ultimate guide to achieving
wholeness. Covering mental and physical health in depth, this book
is a one-stop shop for holistic wellness. Dive in and apply its
wisdom to your life to experience true well-being.*"

— **Pastor Shep Crawford**, Grammy award–winning producer and songwriter

"*Valentina takes you by the hand and leads you through a profound journey
of health transformation.* Well Being *is a moving and empowering guide,
filled with insights and tools that lead you to rewrite the story of your own
health. A must-read if you've ever faced or are facing a health challenge!*"

— **Irene Pace**, food relationship specialist and author of *Eat Like You Teach*

"*I had a front row seat to Valentina's personal transformation.
She courageously navigated some pretty rough seas—taking the road
less traveled, relentlessly committed to facing her fears with Olympic-level
strength, grace, and humility. In* Well Being, *Valentina passionately shares
her journey, with the intention to inspire you to overcome your challenges
and live the life you imagine. I am beyond proud of her and
can't wait for you to benefit from this amazing book!*"

— **Mitch Gaylord**, Olympic Gold Medalist, gymnastics

"If you have found yourself with a copy of Well Being, your journey of self-healing and self-discovery has already begun. Valentina's personal story is raw, honest, and inspiring, divulging immense insight and tools to heal and truly follow one's own path if you have the courage. This book is brave, bold, and beautiful"

— **Kellie Blaise**, actress and writer

"Valentina is a kind, warm, passionate, and aspirational woman, and this is candidly reflected in this book. A true depiction of one's courage and unwavering belief to heal."

— **Lorenzo Agius**, photographer

"I admire Valentina's inner strength and resolve to persevere until she found answers for her healing. Her story is a wonderful, motivating guide. May it reach the hearts and minds of all those who face a struggle like hers and need support."

— **Cathy Rigby**, theater producer, actress, speaker, and Olympic gymnast

"Well Being isn't just a book—it's a lifeline, a beacon of hope, and a guide to reclaiming wellness on every level. Valentina's insights into mental, emotional, spiritual, and physical wellness are profound. Her advice isn't just theoretical; it's practical, actionable, and most importantly, it works. Her warmth and sincerity shine through every page, making the experience both comforting and empowering."

— **Peter Rafelson**, producer, music publisher, and president of Rafelson Media

"Thank you, Valentina, for bringing us a much-needed 'if-I-knew-then-what-I-know-now' book with Well Being. Sharing this type of knowledge could quite literally save someone's life."

— **Randi L. Chapman, MBA**, athlete branding

"Valentina shows us the power of transformation and also how all aspects of us (mind, body, soul) are one. This is a must-read for everyone. She openly shares her own story, which is both touching and inspiring, and I found her wellness journey informative and eye-opening and couldn't put it down until I finished it, staying awake all night."

— **Triona Sheeran**, therapist, QHHT level 3, consciousness speaker

well
being

Published in the United States by: Hay House LLC: www.hayhouse.com˙
Published in Australia by: Hay House Australia Publishing Pty Ltd: www.hayhouse.com.au
Published in the United Kingdom by: Hay House UK Ltd: www.hayhouse.co.uk
Published in India by: Hay House Publishers (India) Pvt Ltd: www.hayhouse.co.in

Cover design: Jason Gabber
Interior design: Bryn Starr Best
Indexer: J S Editorial LLC

Cataloging-in-Publication Data is on file at the Library of Congress

Hardcover ISBN: 978-1-4019-7737-5
E-book ISBN: 978-1-4019-7738-2
Audiobook ISBN: 978-1-4019-7739-9

10 9 8 7 6 5 4 3 2 1
1st edition, October 2024

Printed in the United States of America

This product uses responsibly sourced papers and/or recycled materials.
For more information, see www.hayhouse.com.

well being

A Story of *Healing*
from Autoimmune Disease
and a Guide to Charting
Your Own Path to *Wellness*

Valentina Gaylord

HAY HOUSE LLC
Carlsbad, California • New York City
London • Sydney • New Delhi

I soulfully dedicate this book to you, honoring your journey of healing, enlightenment, transformation, and, beyond all, the beautiful Universe within you.

CONTENTS

INTRODUCTION

A Journey of Transformation

Hello and welcome to *Well Being*! Since this book has found its way to you, know that transformation has already commenced within your very being, heart, soul, and body. You have begun the courageous journey toward whole-body healing, self-discovery, and transformation. Know that you are not alone. You are safe and protected throughout this process of reawakening into your purest and most beautiful form, a fulfillment far greater than you have envisioned for yourself or experienced before now.

This journey is a deep dive within all aspects of your being where transformation is necessary for you to evolve into the person you know you can be—in fact, the person you already are but have kept hidden from yourself and those around you for too long. Your soul has been trying to get your attention in every way imaginable, and you have finally conceded. You are now surrendering to your truth.

Whether your attention has finally been captured by illness, loss, grief, trauma, depression, anxiety, heartbreak, or simply a longing within you for more . . . *you made it here*. These brave new steps forward into your *WELL BEING* will transform your life in ways you cannot foresee, but you will be forever grateful to yourself for doing this work now. Your life ahead will be your greatest adventure—a life free from all that has shattered you before now, and a life transformed that will in turn transform others. You were born with infinite wisdom, innate knowledge, and inherent intelligence, and this book will guide you back to them in ways that will come naturally to you . . . as they were made to and meant to.

With the insight you'll gain as you read this book, you will see into the life you once led with a new perspective. You will look at the circumstances that brought you to this point with an understanding of the greater meaning behind them. With love, respect, honor, and understanding, you will transcend these circumstances and find your way to a place within your being that will feel more like home. This feeling of *home* is powerful, magical, and enchanting, as you will soon come to see, feel, and experience.

I can say this with certainty because I've made this same transformation in my own life—as I'll share with you in the chapters ahead. In my own journey, I extracted illness from my body and self-doubt, limiting beliefs, and unworthiness from my mind for good. I healed my emotional body from loss, grief, trauma, and heartbreak. And I allowed my heart and soul to light my way forward into a life beyond my greatest expectations, desires, and imagination.

I want this for you.

What You'll Find in This Book

Within the pages of this book, I will take you on a transformative journey of whole-body wellness. Together, we will deep-dive into your truth (your story), face your fears, heal your body, and transform your life so you can find meaning, happiness, and abundance within it. You do not need anything outside of yourself to do this work. It is already within you. This work is about being conscious of your subconscious and all you are not allowing to come through to you, that which you are avoiding and suppressing. You have this ability, this light, and this gift within you to make these changes. They are just hidden underneath layers of your past that we will soon discover, uncover, resolve, remove, shift, and rediscover. I will guide you back to your *WELL BEING* with each page you turn.

In Part I, I will share with you my story, and I'll help you start to write *your* story, to find the clarity within it and discern the lessons it is trying to teach you. This is an essential part of your journey, as it holds the secrets and magic you cannot yet see that will form the foundation of your new state of being.

In Part II, we will delve into your *mental wellness*. We will examine your *mindset* to find all the parts of your story that need light, healing, and rewriting of untruths you have been telling yourself. We will open you up to your *intuition* so that you can acknowledge your inner guidance and the truth within you, and then come to a place of *acceptance* of all that has been and will be. This will grant you the *courage* to move forward and face yourself fearlessly and without judgment.

Part III will dive into your *emotional wellness*, where we will heal your emotional body with love and understanding. Starting with *grace*, you will learn the importance of loving yourself, not only in the ways of self-care we all need but in a deeper sense as well. We will discuss *healing, forgiveness, trauma,* and the events that shape our lives, with a focus on understanding the process and overcoming the pain. We will conclude this section with *love*—exploring the valiant heart and the relationships that shape our lives.

From emotional wellness, Part IV will move into *spiritual wellness*, diving into your *beliefs* so you understand there is more to your life and your being than what you can physically see, feel, hear, and touch. We will discuss *meditation* and the messages within that want to be heard by you. Then, my favorite topic, *connection* and how to truly experience both oneness and togetherness, as they are both essential and closely related within your existence. And finally, the ultimate act of love, *surrender*—releasing your past to embrace your present.

As you move through each chapter of this book, you will see, feel, and experience all the benefits of doing this work. Your transformation will happen so quickly, and it will last . . . *a lifetime.* By the time you arrive at Part V, *physical wellness*, you will be ready to take on your *body*, which will have already begun to transform as you've moved through the book. We will discuss *powering* your body, including breaking through the physical and feeling aspects of emotional eating. We will get to know your body *from the inside out* and explore how to safely take on its new form. We will then end in *rest*, which is imperative for living a healthy, happy, balanced, and harmonious life. You will love this chapter if you are a chronic insomniac like I was!

How My Journey Led Me Here

The journey you'll take through this book, as I've just described, has been my journey as well. My life has been transformed in beautiful and undeniable ways because of it, and yours will be too.

My journey unfolded over the course of a decade, beginning with the onset of an autoimmune illness that was repeatedly misdiagnosed and continuing after all traditional medicine, health, and wellness approaches were exhausted. I came to realize that the illness was caused by circumstances I had been avoiding, which were amplified by my relentless drive to help people uncover the mysteries of illness, healing, connection, and happiness . . . *myself included*.

My quest began by founding and building a successful business. I built three award-winning personalized fitness studios over 10 years. At first I believed that physical wellness was the answer I sought and the key to well-being. But I realized early on it was not. After dealing with my own health issues and life's many challenges and working with over 15,000 people, mostly women, who walked through my doors, I realized the physical was only one element of *WELL BEING*, and one that could not work without the others. The mental, emotional, spiritual, and physical elements of wellness had to work together and in wholeness. As a founder, CEO, business owner, entrepreneur, writer, holistic health coach, fitness expert, wife, and mother, I knew I had to bring these elements all together within my own life, my own being, before I could share this journey with my clients—and now with you.

During this time, I continued to educate myself, focusing my mission and my passion on knowledge, research, and seeking the truth that would heal my mind, heart, soul, and body. I profoundly found this truth, and now I can share this life-changing experience with you.

With each day, I am grateful to all those shattered pieces of me that once were, as they brought me to this place. My journey to this place was merciless and tumultuous but necessary to save myself from a life of pain, illness, failure, frustration, and emotional deprivation. It began because it had to, following the shocking diagnosis that forced a reckoning deep within me, a realization that if I did nothing, I would fail not just myself but the family I had built and given my whole heart to.

Untangling the significant impacts of autoimmune disease was just the beginning for me. It demanded an evolution of my mind, heart, soul, and body. My reawakening took over a decade. Yours will not. In the chapters ahead, I will share my story with you and ask you to dive deep within your being to write your own story. At the end of each chapter, please pause, reflect on the questions I pose to you, and look for your own answers within yourself. In this way, you'll transform with me by your side.

You have already proven that you are bold, brave, beautiful, and ready to surrender to an extraordinary life and all that the Universe has waiting for you . . . so, together, let's rekindle your light, reconnect you to your soul, and allow your transformation to take hold.

You will be forever grateful that you did.

• • •

part I

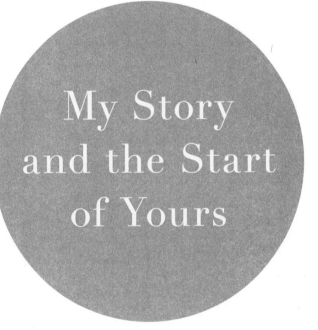

My Story
and the Start
of Yours

Chapter One

THE WAKE-UP CALL COMES

But blind to former as to future fate,
what mortal knows his pre-existent state?

— ALEXANDER POPE

We all have our Part One. This part is the most important, as it holds our journey's hidden gems and secrets, the lessons we came here to learn. They are meaningful and monumental in many ways; they are truly here to guide us, not to hinder us as we so easily assume they are. These are the events that form the cornerstones of our lives. They are the walls we continue to build and hit, time and again, until we realize that we must take action to get beyond the various blockages we have manufactured for ourselves. This journey within is your safe place, a place where you can come to terms with all that you keep hidden within you so that you can release and move past it. This is where your walls will begin to come down in the ways that are truly best for you.

As you read about how my story unfolds, listen to what comes up for you. The feelings, emotions, reflections, and chills you will experience during this chapter are very important pieces of your Part I that we will dive into at the end of this chapter.

How My Part One Began

Bell's palsy was the thruster engine that propelled me toward a wake-up call on March 29, 2012, when I stepped out of the shower.

At that time, I was in global wealth management with two small children: Luc was just under two, and Valletta was just over three.

We were new to Texas and living in North Fort Worth. After living in Malibu and Newport Beach for the last 22 years, we had much to acclimate to: the landscape, the people, our new lifestyle, and a new career. I was 42 years old and, by all measures, in great shape, albeit a bit pinched for time and short on relaxation.

My days had a rigid rhythm to them: up at 4 A.M.; plan the day for myself, my children, and their nanny; hit the gym; shower; and get to work at either my Fort Worth or my Dallas office. After a full day, including an hour sitting in traffic, I would return home for a late dinner with my family, get the children bathed and in bed, make sure our home was meticulously clean, and review all the activities planned for the next day. Yes, I was that person—a complete perfectionist to a significant fault, keeping myself in constant motion, an overachiever avoiding all the deeply rooted issues and emotions I had been diligently suppressing. I was merely existing in life rather than engaging in it. My days were long, nights short, and chronic-stress levels always peaking. But this was the pace I had known since the tender age of seven, when I began to work as a child model for Bonwit Teller and Saks Fifth Avenue—always seeking more, and always outside of myself. My work and working hard was all I knew; it was how I prioritized my goals, dreams, and happiness.

Then, that March morning, everything about my body, process, lifestyle, and future changed. I stepped out of the shower with my husband, Mitch, nearby. As I toweled off from the shower, my left arm suddenly felt heavy. And then numb. Pain, sharp as a lightning bolt, shot through my left ear and the left side of my face. In the foggy mirror, I saw the exterior impact of what was happening inside me. Half my face was drooping, and I couldn't feel the left side of my mouth, the left side of my face, or raise my left eyebrow. I tried to smile, blink, and close my eyes . . . no response. The left half of my face was numb, as though it had detached from the right side and frozen like a separate piece of my body.

I couldn't form words; confusion rocked my brain. As Mitch tried to understand my slurred speech, disoriented state, and sudden physical disabilities, he knew I desperately needed help. We were brand new to the area, unsure where the nearest hospital was, but we knew we had to get there. Being intensely private and willfully stubborn, I did not want to call 911, since that might startle our children or new neighbors from their peaceful sleep. Instead, with our children and their nanny asleep, Mitch bundled me into the car and we set out for a hospital. Thirty minutes later, we found one, and tests began immediately to find out what had happened to shake my good health and life and regimented schedule right off their carefully laid foundation.

• • •

When the doctor on call the next day entered my room, I was coming off a sleepless night of pain, emotional distress, panic, and overthinking. I had overanalyzed myself to prepare for the worst case, the scenario that would take from me everything I had worked my entire life for: my family, career, and life as I knew it and wished it to be.

"You have Bell's palsy," the doctor said.

Horrible projections filled the small hospital room as the doctor talked: the pain and numbness on the left side of my face might never get better, or if it did, it could happen again. When he ordered an MRI, my heart sank even deeper. It took three attempts to squeeze me, a person with claustrophobia, into a tube with mere inches separating the machine from my skin. By then, I was too exhausted to protest any longer, and I recall the extraordinary kindness of the neurologist and nurses who, somehow, got me through it.

The MRI confirmed our worst fears: Bell's palsy was the official diagnosis, and I had suffered brain damage. From that moment, my life began to change.

My first hurdle was preparing my children for what their mother suddenly looked like. What would they do when they saw me? Would I frighten them with a paralyzed face and my inability to smile? My face typically lit up when Valletta and Luc were near; my smile pulled back so widely that my face ached. This brilliant and bright love was all they had ever known from me. At that moment, I knew, above all, I had to make sure my children were okay—even as I was far from it. Our nanny—who was family to us—prepped our children for my return as best she could. Mom was coming home, she told them, but she had gone through something serious, and everyone would work together to help her get better.

As we stopped at a nearby pharmacy to gather my new pre-scriptions, something happened that has affected me deeply every day since. Standing in line, I felt a hand that was not my husband's land gently on my shoulder. A woman, a stranger, standing behind me, bowed her head and began to pray for me. I then watched all 10 people in line behind us place their hands on the shoulders of the person in front of them, dip their chins, and follow her lead in prayer. I felt my soul fill with gratitude as tears flooded my eyes. The stress of my abrupt illness, years of battling chronic worry and anxiety, and my expectations of success broke through the barri-ers I had built. It was a welcome and much-needed release. As my barriers began to shatter slowly, I surrendered and let myself expe-rience this magical moment as the gift it was. Strangers who came together to lend strength and support to a person in need. As each of them hugged me and continued on through the line, I thanked them, feeling deeply impacted by the generosity of their faith and knowing something much deeper was being presented to me. I was always the supportive one, supporting everyone. I had never allowed people to get that close to me or offer me support. It was magical and unsettling all at the same time. Something about who I was was shifting.

As we left the pharmacy to return home, I fell back into silence. My entire focus shifted to my children. The physical evidence of Bell's palsy was all over my face, and I was bracing myself for their reactions. Since I couldn't close my eyes, the doctor gave me a patch. There was no hiding any of it now. Asking Mitch and our nanny, Ann Marie, to take Valletta and Luc into the family room, I entered our home through another entrance and quietly snuck into our bedroom. There, I sat on my bed, breathing deeply and slowly trying to calm my racing heart. I needed to wrap my arms around my children as much as I knew they needed to see me.

My footsteps into the family room felt heavy but deliberate. I approached the children slowly, but they leaped off their father's lap and ran straight for me. Their arms wrapped around me as I kneeled to embrace them. Valletta told me how beautiful I was while Luc laid his tiny little hands upon my face and began to move it gently—his way of trying to put my face back together for me. He knew I had been hurt, and it was his duty—as my son—to fix it. At that moment, I felt the infinite power of my children to help me heal. To this day, they are my beautiful angels.

But it was an unspeakable start to the journey. The pain on the left side of my face soon became unbearable. Desperate for relief, though it went against my instinct, I took the prescribed medication to find some comfort and ease. Then the work on my recovery began. I longed for information and clarity, but I lost hope after several phone calls with close friends in the medical industry. My mind was becoming foggier with every passing moment. I went online and conducted my own research, uncovering an article detailing acupuncture's effectiveness in helping Bell's palsy patients. Next, I researched the credentials of acupuncturists, how they became certified and qualified to practice, and who were among the best in this field. This led me to discover a top master from Taiwan and then to seek any practitioners who had studied under him who might be living and working near my home. It was a long shot, but I was determined. To my surprise, there was an acupuncturist with a successful 31-year career in Southlake, the same city I lived in! It was one of many miracles that would unfold in my life.

The acupuncturist saw me immediately and told me things about Bell's palsy I had not known. Further, he shared what he could do to help me—an expert in his field but an angel on my path. I considered him a godsend, and much like the prayer warriors at the pharmacy, he remains a fixture in my life and my recovery.

We began six-days-a-week treatments for six weeks straight. I was drained, in endless pain, emotionally wrought, and foggy with details, but he restored my hope and determination. I went every day, as scheduled, and by the third day I started to feel my face slightly. A twinge here or a sharp zap there, 90 percent of my face was physically restored by the end of the six weeks of treatments. I no longer needed straws to eat and drink with, and I stopped slurring my words. Drooling was no longer an issue.

Even though watching my face return to its normal state was exhilarating, I was overwhelmed by the repercussions of this massive rehabilitation. My energy was so low that my limbs felt lagging, my long and thick hair was losing its fullness and began falling out, I could no longer concentrate, and my once-bulletproof memory was full of holes. I slowly became a Post-it note queen. Post-it notes were literally everywhere. They were color-coordinated, which my family would come to expect of me *(smiling).*

As vast gaps of time, places, and events opened up in my head, anxiety roared back in, combined with frustration that sent me spiraling into a deep depression. At times, I could not summon the strength to leave my bed. If I tried, my once-strong and toned legs tingled, my feet felt numb, and I would fall to the floor like a rag doll. Always holding back tears, I realized Bell's palsy was just the onset of something more profound. There was more going on, and I was determined to discover it.

With each new day, I would wake up to new symptoms I had never experienced and did not understand. Overcoming them seemed impossible. Uncertainty consumed me, and for the first time in my life, I was deeply concerned with who I would become. I knew I had to fight through this despair to find that part of me that was still alive and willing to take on this challenge. Even though I felt so alone and scared of what this meant for me, my family, my career, and my future, I had to figure this out . . . somehow. With fingers that felt frozen and trembled with exertion, I pushed through weakness and a loathsome sense of lost control and set out yet again to assemble the knowledge and experts I would need to get back to the life I once lived. What I didn't know then was that my very life and lifestyle had brought me to this place.

This was only the beginning for me. As you'll read in Chapter 2, the miracles arrived and the healing began. With more twists and turns along the way, I found peace, and I found myself. I also realized that my very life had brought me to this place, which in turn led me to heal every area of my life. You will, too.

Your Part One

Writing your story is powerful and beautifully healing.
Releasing it from your body is part of this journey.
Take this moment to realize, embrace, and write your Part One.
I will guide you through it with questions for you to answer honestly.
It is just you and me. You will not be measured by anyone for
facing your truth, healing it, and rediscovering yourself.

With your notebook and pencil or laptop in hand, let's begin.

If you experienced feelings, emotions, reflections, or even chills
while reading this chapter, please write them down.
Give yourself this time to get these emotions, feelings, and reflections
out of your body and onto the page. This is the beginning of your
transformation, and I will be here with you every step of the way.

Write about the story that led you to this book—your Part One.
Begin with your wake-up call. I know you had one, and it is time to dive
deep within it safely. Do you know when it came to the surface, where
you were when it happened, and how it made you feel?
Did you understand at that moment what it was?
Do you understand it now? Sometimes we cannot see
it when it happens; we can only see it when we look back
upon it with an open heart and eyes wide open.

Were there life lessons that were and are still evolving for you from
within this experience? Are these lessons repeating themselves in your life?
Who were, or maybe still are, the key individuals in your story?
What or who might be holding you back?
How do you feel about where you are within this story?

In writing your Part One and uncovering its gifts, healing begins.

Once you have written this part of your story,
please join me in Chapter 2.

Chapter Two

MISGUIDED, MISDIAGNOSED, AND THE TRUTH(S) THAT TRANSFORMED ME

Keep your heart in wonder at the daily miracles of your life.

— KHALIL GIBRAN

Welcome back! I hope you have found the beginning of your story, your Part One, and are relaxing into it with the many truths that you have discovered so far. Now we will go even deeper to uncover even more truths as your transformation unfolds. The middle may have been messy, and the end may have been painful, but the journey will be well worth it. This was true in my journey, as you'll see. Let's continue.

• • •

Over the next two years, I went to some of the country's most reputed doctors and specialists seeking solutions to the complex challenge my health had become, yet I was repeatedly misguided and misdiagnosed. This was when depression took me by surprise. Though I was not a depressed person before the onset of Bell's palsy, nor by nature, I was now becoming more and more hopeless. These doctors, whom I respected, kept telling me that I was depressed and that medication could help me ease these symptoms. *Ease my symptoms?* I thought in disbelief and disappointment. I did not wish to ease my symptoms; I wanted them to vanish from my very being, to be ripped from my body as fast as they had set in. I was unwilling to take medication for something I did not believe I had, nor was I willing to settle for reducing these symptoms in any of the ways these doctors all suggested or prescribed. They did not order blood-work or other tests; they just listened to my long list of symptoms and came to their conclusions, and they all came to the same conclusion: I was depressed. None of these doctors and specialists asked me about my life before this fateful event. They were just eager to prescribe me antidepressants, anti-anxiety medication, and anything else they could confine me to indefinitely without any real evidence of what was wrong. By some of these specialists, I was told I "could" have multiple sclerosis, Parkinson's disease, early-onset dementia, Sjögren's syndrome, lupus, and so on.

So I went on to see more specialists, including neurologists, to have tests and bloodwork done to rule these other ailments out, which I successfully did. Next I turned to functional medicine doctors, well-known nutritionists, naturopaths, healers, and even gurus. I was desperate for answers because nothing anyone had told me resonated within me, and I refused to settle for what was becoming of me. I was desperate, determined, frustrated, and stubborn to a fault. But it seemed the solution from these new specialists, too, was to squeeze me into a one-size-fits-all box and prescribe me even more medications, supplements, and an abundance of hormones . . . and all at once! At one point, I went against all my instincts and succumbed to taking bioidentical medication and 66 supplements daily because I thought maybe, just maybe, my stubborn nature was getting in the way of my healing. That turned out to be true, but not in the way I had originally believed. More on this later *(smiling)*.

Nothing worked, which made me feel even worse than I had felt when this journey began. My body was changing in ways that I could not control, and in the process of losing control, I was losing my self-worth and self-confidence as well. I felt I was losing *myself*, and rapidly. Any hope that things would improve had now escaped me; it was all a smoldering, pressure-filled casket of hopelessness. I was becoming a shell of the person I once was, and I was exhausted, disheartened, and utterly confused.

Then something happened that gave me a flicker of hope. It sparked deep within me while I was visiting one of the last specialists

I would ever see. Something inside of me was trying to get my attention. That was a familiar feeling that I had dismissed so many times before now. This time, though, I was not ignoring it; I was paying attention to it. I am sure you have felt this kind of feeling, and you are probably becoming more aware of them. If not, you soon will.

I was sitting in the office of a highly regarded dermatologist in the city I lived in then. His wife was a physician and a client of mine, so I trusted that I was in good hands. I went to see him because I woke up with redness in the shape of a butterfly on both sides of my cheeks, something I had not experienced before. He took one look at me and diagnosed me with lupus. He did not order bloodwork or tell me to see my primary care physician. He just diagnosed me on the spot in less than one minute with no questions asked and gave me two prescriptions for topical creams. That was it.

My heart sank once again. Did he honestly try to prescribe me medication without any substantial evidence that I did indeed have lupus? Intuitively (thanks to that feeling), and without question, I knew that I did not have lupus, but I needed to be sure that my feeling was accurate. I bolted out of the dermatologist's office and called the physician assistant at my ob-gyn's office. I asked her to order me lab work for lupus straightaway. This PA was incredible during this time. Every time I was diagnosed (or misdiagnosed, rather) with something, she and I would work together to rule it out. She ordered the test for me before we ended our call, so I drove straight to the lab and had the test done. Then I went home and began doing some research of my own. The test would take 48 hours to return results, so I began to process this experience. I felt there was a much deeper meaning behind it, and I was slowly opening up to the meaning and to what my body was trying to tell me.

Even so, I found myself going outside of myself once again, turning to the Internet instead of my own intuitive guidance. For symptom checks, I always turned to the Mayo Clinic, WebMD, and Healthline for information, so this is what I did once again. Astonishingly enough, I found that the redness on my cheeks could be a vitamin B deficiency. *Could it be that simple?* I thought. I then researched foods with vitamin B and found a list—most of which

I loved but had not had in quite some time—so I went straight to the grocery store and loaded up on broccoli, Brussels sprouts, chickpeas, sweet peas, and Siggi's yogurt (dessert in a cup) and planned to incorporate these foods into my meals over the following week to see if that was all my body needed to eliminate the redness from my face. I was already eating a plant-based diet, but now I focused on these foods primarily.

Meanwhile, the lupus test came back negative, and within one week of incorporating these foods, the redness in my cheeks was gone. My body had, in fact, been deficient in vitamin B. That feeling I had in the doctor's office was absolutely correct.

This was the beginning of so much more to come. Looking back, I can see how the butterfly-shaped redness on my cheeks symbolized the transformation that would soon come for me. I didn't yet understand that it was my life that needed a complete overhaul and that my body was just its messenger—but that epiphany was coming soon.

Now, two years in, on the brink of my 44th birthday, with no real answers but armed with some new insight, I asked myself some serious questions: What did I want for my life, health, career, family, and future? What was I most unhappy with? What could I control? And more importantly, what could I change? I made a list. A very, very, very long list. At the very top was regaining my strength and good health. Just below that, a change of scenery (my BIG move to Paris, France, that I had postponed numerous times) and a new career path based on holistic health and wellness and finding answers where there were none. This was now at the forefront of my life. I knew that once I helped myself, I wanted to help others going through the same thing. But it had to happen in that order. I had to live through this, find my way back to great health, and restore my life. I had to find the answers to what plagued me—and also plagued many others, as I was beginning to see.

So I focused on my physical body, once again looking outside myself for the answers.

Before we moved to Texas in 2011, we lived in Southern California. In those days, I worked out two to four hours daily and was incredibly healthy and health-conscious, or so I thought. Now that I was no longer in a position to do that in my newfound life and health crisis in Texas, I began strategizing how I could build something in its place—how I could create an environment in Texas that housed some of the things I loved so much about my workouts in California, minus my running, as that was something I could no longer do. As I slowly regained function and mobility, I developed a workout routine that fit my life as both a career-driven mom and someone still very much in recovery from an illness no one knew how to name or cure. My workouts were far removed from what they once were, but I knew I had to start somewhere and move my body more and more with each day, even when I did not want to, which was most days. While I recognized I no longer had the energy, stamina, or time I'd had before, I still coveted the way I felt during my California days. I longed for those days and needed to return them to my life somehow. With that in mind, after a lot of planning, and a move from North Fort Worth to Austin, Texas, I opened my first personalized fitness studio, a boutique studio that was unlike any other I had been to before. I wanted to do something no one else was doing, something with the potential to reach people struggling as profoundly as I had been and still was. Something that would help me heal while I helped others achieve their fitness goals. Coming from a corporate background with a newfound passion for health and wellness, a fitness studio seemed the best way to start.

Austin wasn't the BIG move to Paris that I had been planning all of my life, but I made do . . . once again. In Austin, I launched my first boutique fitness studio. This gave me the physical environment that I thought I needed to look ahead at an even bigger vision: a company that would eventually evolve into a holistic health-and-wellness brand that would support a full spectrum of life-changing experiences for my clients, community, and team—support that I had not received, but that I could offer others.

Then a drama began that turned my good intentions into the nightmare—or nightmares, plural—that would shake me into submission and form the person I am today. I fought it every step of

15

the way. Instead of surrendering to the Universe, I worked against it, and the lessons that came were devastating but ultimately woke me up to my truth.

Here is what happened. Shortly after I opened my first studio, I was approached by an investor who came in to take a class. He was a respectable and very wealthy businessman—in fact, a billionaire—at the time, and I believed him to be trustworthy. Eager to expand my brand and grow it to the vision that I intended, I went into partnership with him. Still struggling with my health, I found a way to manage the merger with absolute certainty that it was the right move forward.

My only major concern, a gut feeling that turned out to be completely accurate, was about his wife. Gut feelings are meant to guide us. Avoiding them never ends well, as you will come to see. This man was married to a woman who was not as honorable as he was, at least not by my standards. It was the only thing I ever questioned about him, but my eagerness to grow my business surpassed my gut feeling when I met her. She was not part of the partnership, which made me feel confident in overlooking my qualms. I had worked with many billionaires worldwide throughout my career in private equity, and none of them ever allowed their spouses to interfere with their business partnerships, so I assumed he was of the same mindset.

I opened two more studio locations back-to-back within the first two and a half years. I felt hopeful during this period of rapid growth, but it also brought some of the hardest lessons of my life. Work demands were intense, which I was used to, but my body was continuing to shut down on me. This mysterious illness my body was battling remained unmanageable and, at times, completely debilitating. I used every ounce of strength I had to forge through it, as I always had, not realizing the powerful messages that my body was trying to convey to me.

As my 46th birthday neared, I contemplated the year ahead—after four years of misdiagnoses and no real answers or relief. I was working nonstop, bringing my vision to life while chained to a burdensome, baffling condition that sapped my energy and yanked apart my existence. While I had good moments, I was withering away, and I recognized I could no longer continue this way. Intuitively, I remained convinced I was missing the most significant turning in the labyrinth that would lead me back to wellness.

Nothing in my family history that hails from the Mediterranean and Europe is genetically linked to illnesses like this. As relatives from Malta, France, London, Australia, Ibiza, and Italy started reaching out to wish me a happy birthday and new year, I used the opportunity to dive deeper into my lineage. I identified a few cases of cancer, including my father, aunt, and uncle. I wondered if I, too, had some form of cancer that the specialists had missed. Having been immersed in physical cataclysms for so long, I often feared the worst. At this stage, I even began thinking about estate planning for my business and making plans for the ongoing care of our children should something happen to me. It seemed a logical and yet heartbreaking necessity during this time.

Though my business was growing and evolving, ignoring my initial gut feelings about my business partnership proved disastrous. I found myself in a two-year arbitration centered on my business partner and his wife, an unimaginable betrayal by individuals I should have been able to trust within the establishment I had built from the ground up. People I generously gave opportunities to by hiring them, training them, and trusting them within the walls of my business. Stress levels were at an all-time high for me, which caused even more setbacks with my health. This was not why I set out on this journey, but it was teaching me life-altering lessons through all the pain, disappointments, betrayals, and setbacks. I was humbled, disarmed, and dismantled so that I could become the person I am today. Looking back now, I realize that this was the greatest gift this time in my life gave to me.

I had to stay focused on getting through it all amid the chronic fatigue and brain fog that did not lift. I focused solely on saving the business I had worked hard to build and sacrificed so much for. I was resolute in removing atrocious people from my business and my life while keeping the people on my team who deserved to be there and keeping my community thriving. It was a challenging few years, since I trusted no one after this. But I was determined and willing to see this through while my health was privately, and unbeknownst to anyone other than my family, continuing to decline.

Then something miraculous happened. One day while I was scrolling on Facebook, something I had rarely done before, a book advertisement kept popping up on my page. That feeling appeared in my life once again. I knew I had to read this book, and then it was as if something outside of me, a force much greater than I, moved my finger to click on it without my permission or assistance. The book was *Medical Medium* by Anthony William. Without question, I ordered it. It was Friday morning, January 1. The book was set to be delivered by Sunday, January 3, my birthday, which I saw as yet another sign that this book was coming into my life for a significant reason and purpose. I was overflowing with excitement and promise, something I had not felt in over four years.

As it turned out, the book arrived not within two days, but within two hours. It was New Year's Day, and there the book was, lying on my front doorstep. To this day, I wish I could have thanked and hugged the person who delivered this book to me. They delivered something to me that would change the course of my life, only I did not know it at the time. I was just in awe, as it felt so personalized and just for me. I began reading it within minutes. I stayed home all weekend and read this book from cover to cover. Laid out within the pages was everything I had felt, sensed, and lived through over the past several years symptomatically. Suddenly, profound hope arose inside me, and I knew I had to speak to Anthony. I had to understand the truth about what was happening to me, and it felt as though he might hold the answers when no one else did.

On the morning of my 46th birthday, I woke up with a clarity that had escaped me for years. Now was the time to exchange all my confusion, pain, and misery for a new trajectory. I sat in contemplation and considered everything I had ever truly loved and needed, what was working, what was not, and what and who had failed me the most. Then I decided to change it all. I would create a plan and then strategically accomplish it. I had been a natural multitasker before the onset of my illness, but now I knew I would need to take each step with undivided attention to its every detail.

I had a call with Anthony William four weeks later. I wanted to get to the heart of my health issues and overcome them, as I believed they were the root cause of all my symptoms. In the days leading up to our call, I felt an anxious expectation. Could he possibly deliver me the news that I so desperately needed? I knew I needed to remove all doubt and replace it with concrete answers. I knew I needed to explore Anthony's gifts to find out what was causing my symptoms and surrender to his words, whatever they might be. He was my last hope of finding answers when all else had failed me. I braced for the possibility of him delivering bad news about my health but felt ready to accept whatever was coming my way.

• • •

The morning of the call, I was calm until I heard Anthony's voice. It was tranquil and soothing, and yet I felt suddenly unprepared to listen. I prattled on with nonsensical musings in some form of defense mode to prevent him from informing me of how dire my future would be. With his kind and gentle nature, Anthony broke through all that chatter, calming me down and preparing me to receive what he offers as a medium.

While silently skeptical and nervous, I also wanted to be open and respectful of his gift and his time. Anthony knew nothing about me before our call; I wanted this to be a genuine experience I could trust. It was precisely that.

As Anthony started talking about my health, I relaxed, and my body exhaled. It was as if I had been holding my breath until that moment.

Once I let my guard down, his intuitive reasoning delivered an answer quite shocking to me: *Epstein-Barr virus (EBV)*. Anthony told me I had the virus in my liver and thyroid. He told me to have my doctors run a blood test to confirm it and to also perform an ultrasound on both my liver and thyroid. Yet another new path had emerged. Could it be, at long last, the answer I sought?

Anthony's simple suggestions included eating a plant-based diet for a period of time so that my body could heal—easy, given that I was already following one—along with taking supplements.

He added in daily celery juice, fruit, and specific vegetables, and suggested removing certain foods as well. He predicted I would be off thyroid medication within three years. In four years and consultations with the best doctors in the country, none had ever uncovered what Anthony revealed to me . . . and over the phone! Anthony also discussed Valletta and Luc, even though I had not previously mentioned my children to him. With his gift, Anthony knew of them both and knew that they suffered from severe anaphylactic food allergies. He provided a plan for them too, something tangible that could be helpful if future reactions were to occur. My half-hour call had stretched into one hour and a long-lasting friendship—it was one of the absolute best hours of my life.

Once the call was over, I called my current doctor, because I now needed to confirm these new findings, and asked for an ultrasound of my liver and thyroid and a blood test for EBV. Shockingly enough, these tests had never been ordered or even mentioned by any of the many doctors I had seen up to this point. Two hours later, I was having blood drawn. Twenty-four hours later, I learned my thyroid had a nodule, my liver had suffered damage from medications and supplements I had never needed, and I did have Epstein-Barr virus in my liver and thyroid. Anthony was right!

As I began to follow Anthony's suggestions, I intuitively knew that I had to go even deeper. My symptoms began to dissipate and resolve themselves over the next few months, giving me the mental clarity to begin to develop a stronger mindset and a more purposeful mission. My once rapidly waning energy was now brimming with sustained stamina that fed my renewed creativity. My mind could retain new information and produce memories I had feared were gone forever. My life was returning to me, and it was the most exciting feeling I have had in nearly a decade!

Still, I had many unanswered questions. I had a clear and trusted pathway to restoring my health, but now I needed to know the why behind my illness. I needed to understand in order to ensure that it would never return in the form I had experienced—or in an even worse form from which I could not recover. What brought it on? What caused this major turn of events that in mere seconds took away my health for nearly a decade? What was my body trying to tell me, and when did it begin? What was it about my life that brought me to this place?

I would soon find out.

The next seven years played out like a nightmare I could not wake up from. The two-year arbitration, followed by the COVID-19 pandemic, was absolutely brutal on me and my business. My health was vacillating throughout it all. My stress levels were beyond my control, and sleep deprivation was all I knew. I felt like a shell of a person moving robotically through my life as it played out before me in slow motion. My walls were up higher than they had ever been, and I was lost in all that was happening around me. This life that I was living was so far from where it all began. The hope, the joy, the vision, and the passion for all that I set out to create when I ventured into this endeavor—these were lost, and so was I.

In 2022, at age 52, I was gutted. I felt that my life as I knew it was over. It was a time of absolute heartbreak, include the passing of my father and the sale of my business.

And yet, this was when this work came to fruition. My life did not end there as I so dramatically believed it had *(smiling)*. It began.

I dove deep within my being, my experiences, and my life, and I found myself. I found the truth. I found my soul, a version of myself that I had deeply felt existed for me, but that I was too afraid to access. I always felt that if I did, my world as I knew it would end. It ended anyway, despite my many efforts to hold tightly on to it, and it was the best thing that ever happened to me. It will be for you too.

My life is what made me sick. What I thought was happiness became my demise. None of it brought me the happiness I believed it would—or that I feel now. My body was my wake-up call because all the little signs along the way were ignored.

This story is mine, but shared and fortified by so many. The work you complete in this book will be revealed upon the surface of your life, but it begins deep within you, as it did with me. The path to healing is by healing all of you. It goes beyond the physical into the mental,emotional, spiritual, and physical aspects of your life and being.

Your Part One, Continued

*This part of your story takes
vulnerability and the truth. Your truth.*

*Please be brutally honest with yourself and mindful of your
feelings as you write this part of your story. Allow yourself this safe
place and space to express yourself as you answer these questions . . .
without judgment. Releasing these emotions from your
body is essential to your healing journey.*

*We all have a vision for our lives that begins
when we are children, when we are most innocent
and untainted from the world that surrounds us now.
It changes throughout our lives, but one theme
always stays with us. What was that for you?*

*Can you remember when your life began to feel uneasy, stressful,
fearful, and not aligned with your hopes, truth, and dreams?
When did that begin, and when did that end for you?
How did the ending make you feel? Did you feel misguided,
misled, manipulated, betrayed, misdiagnosed, or judged?
Express all those feelings here.*

Did you or do you feel alone or unsupported in this journey?

*Have you had gut or intuitive feelings that you followed
that proved to be accurate? Have you had gut or intuitive feelings that
you did not follow that proved to be accurate? How did they make you
feel when you followed them and when you did not?*

Have you experienced miracles in your life? Do you believe in them?

Miracles are coming. Let's get you ready to embrace them.

*As soon as you are ready, let's journey through your
transformation together, beginning with your **mindset**.*

part 11

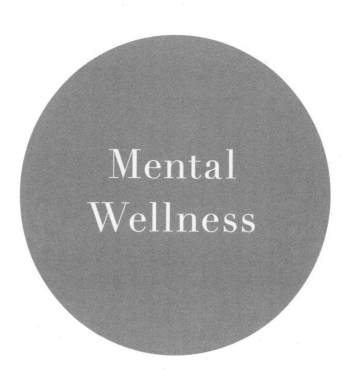

Mental
Wellness

Chapter Three

MINDSET

The Stories We Tell Ourselves

*Our anxiety does not come from thinking about the future,
but from wanting to control it.*

— KHALIL GIBRAN

Bell's palsy and the diagnosis of Hashimoto's that I ultimately received were my catalysts for change. When nothing else could get my attention, my body became my beacon, guiding me home from the storm. Food was the medicine that reversed my ailments and relieved me of my symptoms, but it was the lifestyle changes I knew deep within I had to make that brought me to this place, living the life that I truly desired. It was doing this work that brought me vibrantly back to life, mind, heart, soul, and body.

Woven within the depths of your story is your truth. Now that you have a much deeper understanding of your story, where it began, and how you arrived here, let's dive deep within your soul to discover, heal, and transform all the aspects of your life that brought you here with clarity. Facing these truths now may feel uncomfortable at first, but it will change your life in the most beautiful and profound ways.

If your walls are up and your armor is intertwined with each fiber of your body, as mine was before doing this work, I ask that you allow these walls to come down so that together we can release all the chains that bind you to a life that no longer supports you.

It begins with your mindset.

Your mind and your intuition are your most powerful gifts of consciousness. When in collaboration, your life is boundless. When in dissonance, your life is bound. The beauty of this is that it is your choice.

Your mind (mindset), when in alignment with your soul (intuition), will orchestrate with you and bring harmony and balance to your life. When in discord, it will work against you, mislead you, and deceive you by focusing on who you once were and who you might become based on your past efforts and missteps, viewing these in the light of something you did wrong versus the lessons they came into your life to teach you. In this place of disconnection, it is impossible to see your way forward with clarity. This is where we become frozen in time; our lives become stagnant, and unhappiness sets in. Living in this space bound by negative thought patterns and their many deceptions, we become disconnected from ourselves in ways that relinquish our joy, happiness, and purpose, not just now but for the unforeseen future. Shifting your mindset allows your life to truly emerge in the way that it was meant to.

In embracing your mindset, an essential aspect of your spiritual body, you will gain mastery over your life by becoming conscious of these unconscious thought patterns that have played out in your mind and controlled you for far too long. This may seem difficult or impossible to achieve, but it is not. If I can learn to quiet my mind, so you can you *(smiling)*. Before now, I was an overachiever at overthinking and overanalyzing everything to the point of nausea. The work we are doing here will bring you the clarity and peace that you need to persevere and prosper, especially if illness or inner conflict exists within your life presently.

Mastering your mindset is the foundation of your whole body transformation, as it will open up all the beauty and all the magic that is here and waiting for you. It is the key to unlocking your intuition. Your intuition, like health, is your birthright, your saving grace. Your inner sanctuary, oneness within, and the knowingness that is home to your soul's purpose and energy force. A place where inspiration, passion, love, truth, joy, *well-being*, health, happiness, and forgiveness flourish. Your mindset is a powerful force that wants you to take the lead, not by trying to control it but by trying to understand it. It is with understanding that you will learn to master it.

Our mindset is, in a way, meant to derail us until we become conscious of this and then learn how to transcend it. We believe it is our truth when it is not. It is all based on our own fears—fears of the truth and the change that the truth will bring us, good or not so good. Acknowledging this, and understanding that it all comes from fear and not love, is where we can begin to heal this very important part of ourselves.

I have come to refer to it as the subterfuge mind, aka the ego, the deceptive mind. We all have one, and it challenges us all. I know this to be true for you, too, and you are not alone. You already know this voice; it is that inner critic that is not in union with your intuition, the one that deceives you into believing you are not worthy of the meaningful and tangible things in life that your soul desires and deserves. You may already be consciously trying to silence this inner critic. If you are, that is a brave and bold step in the right direction.

Becoming the Observer

One of the most unequivocal ways of silencing this critical observer is by observing its critiques as they pass through your mind without judgment, allowing them to come through as they are. Continuing to judge yourself by them will only lead you back down the path that brought you here. You are not going that way *(smiling)*. This time, move through the critiques in a different way. Observe how they make you feel, and feel into them. Allow yourself to really feel the feelings as these thoughts pass through your mind and body, without avoiding or suppressing them, so that you can release them from your body. I know these might be difficult feelings for you to sit with, but processing these feelings and emotions is the only way to bring light to them, heal them, and ensure they leave your thoughts and your body forever—which they will.

Observe these thoughts, the meaning you place on them, and where they came from. Are these recurring themes in your life? Is there a lesson in these thoughts that can shed a positive light on your life? By observing these self-criticisms and changing your perception of them, you will find resolution and resolve within them—the lessons. By gently and gracefully rewriting what these thoughts mean to you, you will release the heaviness of carrying them for as long as you have—the weight of the world, so to speak. By "rewriting" them, I do not mean rewriting history. You cannot change your past, but you can change its meaning. This is what I want you to do now. Find the meaning—the hidden truths within your observations, the why behind all that has happened to you before now. The why is the lesson.

Observing the "Other" Stories We Tell Ourselves

You may find that not all of the stories that hold you back are yours, yet you have taken them on as your own. I have seen this pattern repeatedly, mostly in women whom I have worked with throughout my career. There are a few I have heard repeatedly over the last decade that have especially concerned me because I know that women worldwide have taken them to heart and believe them to be true. We can become so programmed to believe something that will only work against us in the bigger picture of our lives— and the reality of these stories is that they are also based on fear, of failure and of change. They can easily be used to create excuses that delay our happiness indefinitely and leave us feeling hopeless and confused. Understanding what might be happening in someone else's reality does not mean it needs to bleed over into yours. Everyone has their own life lessons to work through and in their own time, so if you are holding on to beliefs that do not belong to you, please release them, too.

I will give you an example of a story like this, one you have probably heard before. It is absolutely untrue. I once believed this story to be true for me—at the onset of my illness—so I understand how it feels, but I have personally debunked it in my own life several times.

On a daily basis, I would hear from my new clients—whether they were 25 years old or 75—that their metabolism had slowed down because of childbirth, illness, age, perimenopause, menopause, or postmenopause and that they were "never" going to be able to lose weight or get into great shape ever again. I had several doctors tell me this at different stages of my life. This story is absolutely untrue. But if you believe it, it will become true for you, because you will make it true through the actions that you take that your thoughts have provoked. You will essentially give up. But if you make the appropriate modifications to your nutrition, and exercise your body in a way that benefits you, you will prove this story wrong. I proved it wrong, and many of my clients have done so too. It is a mindset that needs to be shifted so that you can focus on what is really true for you.

If there is a story like this that is running in your mind, know that it has served its purpose in your life and prepare to release it. As you observe and release these themes from your mind, your life will begin to become clear. All that has held you back will come to the forefront of your mind so you can transmute it, release it, and move beyond it. This is a choice. You can either continue to carry it with you or begin to release it. As soon as you release it, your life will begin to take on its new form.

The Release

Once you become conscious of these thoughts that have been repeatedly playing in your mind, you can release them from your body and your life. They will no longer linger, haunt you, or hold you back—as they have for most of your life. Our mindset begins in our youth, at such an early stage in our lives that we may have no recollection of its first occurrence; we only know it has been with us for as long as we can remember. The people and situations in our lives may change, but the patterns and the lessons remain the same until we do the inner work to transform them. We will talk more about this in the coming chapters. Whether or not you can recall the exact moment in your life when you began to have these negative thoughts and perceptions about yourself, it is time to release them. They do not support you in the way that you need to be supported in your life.

Releasing with Gratitude

Releasing these thoughts might feel daunting at first, as you have come to rely on them so heavily and perhaps even hide behind them, as I once did. But the truth is you know now is the time to do this work. That is why you are here, so let's do this together.

It is always best to release these emotions with gratitude for the lessons the patterns have taught you, their importance in your journey, and the way in which you are evolving because of them. At first, this will be something you need to do every day until these thoughts no longer come to the surface of your mind. As you move through each chapter of this book and dive deeper into your healing, you will be able to overcome these thoughts completely and be in harmony with your intuition; that is where the magic and healing in all areas of your life will appear.

When you reach that point—and you will—your life will transform right before your eyes.

The Magnitude of This Journey

The magnitude of my journey toward true happiness, fulfillment, and healing took close to two decades, far longer than it needed to. I unconsciously allowed my inner critic to keep me in a perpetual state of inconsequence where its fear-based undertones and louder-than-life noise silenced my intuition. I was not living my truth; I knew this with every ounce of my being.

Had I had this clarity sooner and been able to listen to my intuition, which was a constant force in my life trying to get my attention, I could have avoided many traumatic events in my life, including the debilitating illness that forced a reckoning within me to do this work. I could have avoided these situations had I trusted my intuition rather than the opposing voice in my mind, my inner critic. I now understand how fear was at the nucleus of it all and how it wielded its power over my thoughts and over me. Once you have this epiphany, and you will, you will be forever free from fear's restraints. I was always a very stubborn person, and I held on to these limiting beliefs for far too long. Once I surrendered to doing this deep inner work, it all changed for me, and it changed rapidly as it will for you too.

Your mindset is potent, and as powerful as it is, you control it—no one else. You have the power over the thoughts you allow to come through to you, how you process these thoughts, and how you dismiss them when necessary, which it will be essential that you do at times—in fact, at most times. It is not as difficult as it may seem right now. It is quite simple once you become conscious of these thoughts. You do this by observing them, accepting them for what they are, and giving power to the beliefs you cherish rather than those you do not. It is a choice. Your choice.

We all have this profound inner critic that moves, defines, shakes, and can quickly destroy us at its whim without us even questioning it. We give this voice so much power over our well-being, especially in times of crisis, stress, anxiety, and fear, when it seems to be a constant force holding us back. This voice will keep you frozen, unmoving, and devoid of all that you truly cherish and desire in life if you continue to allow it to, consciously or unconsciously. So I ask you to start questioning it—really questioning it—now.

After all I had been through, I began observing this inner critic and the thoughts it had created that I had given so much of my power to. I listened to these critiques more openly and intentionally. I felt these thoughts as they flowed across my mind, and I could see them for what they truly were. Then I questioned them. I dove deep within myself to uncover the why behind these thoughts and the inner critic that created them; there was a why, and I was going to find my way to it. Once I reached this point, I knew I would never give these thoughts power over me again.

Think of it this way. Our mindset creates the reality of our thoughts. Our thoughts ignite our beliefs, which become the foundation of our values, empowering our behavior. Your thoughts are powerful, and they become a part of everything that you do and, in turn, affect your overall health and wellness. Once you become aware of this, you can change the pattern of events to work with you rather than against you. You can create a new meaning for your thoughts, especially the reccurring ones.

In my own moments in silence, I asked myself the tough questions I had been avoiding and faced the answers that came to me with an open heart. I gave myself grace. Was there something that had gone unresolved in my life? What part of me held on to self-doubt, shame, or feelings of unworthiness? What was I so drawn to that I was afraid to either pursue or let go of? In my silence, I allowed myself to be open to the messages I received. I resisted resisting them. I now understood the profound difference between the inner critic that created these thoughts and the intuition that would gracefully guide me throughout the rest of my life.

As you begin to observe your inner critic consciously, you will come to understand its place in your life. It is not a humble voice; it needs your attention as it implores you to hear, see, feel, and resolve it. Once you do resolve it, this critic will no longer have any power over you.

It is not only this inner critic that uses its mighty will to derail us. It's also the stories we hear that we take on as our own, as we've seen. The stories that we take on and tell ourselves are the stories that keep us stuck. Much like our inner critic, we hear things we perceive as truth, and then we take them on as our own, using them as excuses for accepting mediocrity versus a fulfilled life. We settle. These stories deprive us of our joy, our love for life, our love for ourselves and others, our happiness, and ultimately, our dreams and ambitions. They remove us from our natural state of consciousness.

Since you have this book within your grasp, you and I both know that you are at a place in your life where genuine transformation is of the essence, and you are prepared to embrace it. You know that you are your soul, your story, your gifts, and your journey, and that is what is true and beautiful for you. Though it will take every ounce of courage, strength, bravery, and discernment and an unwavering commitment to yourself, first and foremost, this new state of consciousness will bring you to your knees in gratitude.

I had thought that I was a conscious person, but my journey toward living a truly conscious life taught me differently. It began with the onset of my illness. I had avoided what I knew to be true; now my body would get my attention when nothing else could, and it did just that. I was bound by it and forced to face its truth. It took courage, strength, and patience to get to where I am today, but I did it, and you will, too.

We are all intuitive. As we evolve, this gift becomes more prominent in our lives. It truly is our saving grace. It was only when I learned how to fiercely silence my inner critic that I could genuinely hear and deeply feel my intuitive guidance beyond any reasonable doubt.

By silencing the opposing voices within you, you will allow *your* intuition to guide you. You will not hinder or sabotage your own path by denying its existence. It is as natural as you are. Your body encapsulates its magic. Only you can set it free to take you where you were born to go.

If I were there with you, I would wrap my arms around you and hug you tightly to support your dauntless gallantry and assure you that you will reach that place. You are laying your pathway there, stone by stone.

Your Mindset

In observing your own mindset, can you see the areas within your life that your inner critic has hindered? Can you clearly see the repeated patterns and stories throughout your life and identify their commonalities? Can you see, with absolute certainty, the lessons in these patterns that have presented themselves time and again?

With grace, love, and understanding, can you release these thought patterns from your mind? Can you sit with them, feel your way through them, and release them from your mind and body?

Can you find a new meaning for them? One that brings you understanding and compassion for who you once were and who you are becoming?

Can you find peace of mind knowing that these thoughts, patterns, and critiques will no longer be a part of your life?

With each day, it will get easier and easier for you to move through these thoughts, feelings, and emotions. Soon, you will arrive at a place where they might enter your mind, but they will not stay as you will quickly move past them with a positive and healthy mindset that will support you in all the ways that make life more fulfilling. A mindset that is in partnership with your **intuition**.

Chapter Four

INTUITION

Acknowledging Your Inner
Guidance and the Truth within You

Trust. Your. Intuition.

Intuition is your superpower. Beyond reason or reservation, it is your saving grace. Your inner compass. Its guidance is your pathway to the life you wish to live. You need nothing more, as there is nothing more powerful than this. All you have to do is listen.

As you begin releasing your mind from the noise that has consumed you all these years, I want you to reflect on the many moments in your life where your intuition has guided you successfully or was proven accurate when you did not follow it. How did these experiences unfold and make you feel? Did you follow through without interference, or did you let your mind interfere? If you allowed interference, these experiences did not go as planned, I am sure. There would have been a lesson or two to learn. If you did follow through without interference, I am sure it unfolded exactly how you felt it would, perhaps even better than you had imagined. Still, valuable lessons are to be learned—in this case, lessons that align with who you are in your heart and soul.

In doing this work, you will find that your mindset is manufactured only in your mind after years, perhaps decades, of programming and conditioning. Your intuition is an instinct, a gut reaction, and a feeling that can only be felt in your heart and soul. It is a gift that you were born with. This is how you know the difference.

When you overcome your current mindset and come into harmony with your intuition, magic and healing in all areas of your life will be inevitable. When you reach this point, your life will transform right before your eyes in ways that transcend anything you could have imagined for yourself. You will witness what has always been waiting for you all this time. You will feel a sense of serenity, an undeniable trust, a sensuous calm, and a peacefulness come over you all at once, and all the noise will cease. You will find yourself more centered, and your ability to follow your heart and your intuition will flow more freely through you. You will genuinely believe in yourself, your abilities, and your desires and begin your mental and emotional healing journey with a newfound sense of purpose and meaning that will stay with you for the rest of your life.

In this moment, you will experience oneness within your heart, soul, and being. With clarity, you will understand all that you had not understood before. All will become clear, and this will unleash your soul's purpose and your energy force right before your eyes. You will feel illuminated and become invincible in your own right. You will begin to see beyond the physical universe you have created for yourself and into the empyreal feeling of where your life is heading. Every fear you have ever had will leave your body, and you will have trust and faith that words alone cannot honestly describe or explain. I know this because it happened to me and will happen to you. It captivated me. It left me breathless. It left me speechless— and I always have much to say *(smiling)*.

I never would have believed this could be possible until it happened to me. The Universe stepped in when I needed it most, and through all the pain, sacrifice, and heartbreak I was feeling at the time, it brought me such solace, only this time, it came through significant changes in my life that I had been avoiding and could avoid no longer. I knew in this moment I had to rein in my thoughts, let go of the meaning they once had for me, and relinquish their power over me. Then I became vulnerable to and in oneness with my intuition. I finally felt aligned, or, shall I say, realigned, as you will see. I will share this next story with you so you can see how living in my mind (ego) brought me so much misery and pain that I could not even feel my successes when I had them. My happiness was diminished, and my light had vanished. Had I listened to intuition, all of this would have been avoided. It was in going against my intuition that my unhappiness flourished. This story will help *you* understand why healing your mindset is so important, because without it, you will not hear your intuition and you will not live in alignment with your truth.

The Beginning of the End—My End

This is the story of my demise *(smiling)*. My life-altering challenges began in late 2016, after years of denying my intuition. They culminated in 2022. The arbitration that began in 2017 ended in late 2019. I was beginning to recover from two horrific years of defending myself and my business from some very dishonorable, even delusional individuals. Fortunately for me, the arbiter saw this lawsuit for what it truly was, and the case against my business ended. It was finally over. I was relieved and exhausted. The year 2020 was before me, and I was looking forward to starting a new year with the arbitration behind me. I was excited . . . for about a minute.

During the years of arbitration, I had been working with new investors to launch a new brand more aligned with the vision I had initially set out to create. We were preparing to meet in Los Angeles on March 14, 2020, to discuss the details. As we prepared to travel to Los Angeles from different parts of the country, some startling news began to surface worldwide. COVID-19 was upon us. As a small business owner, I was terrified, to say the least. Things were changing, and they were changing fast.

My relationship with my current business partner was compromised by the arbitration, so, needless to say, I no longer trusted our relationship. I was determined to save my business again, and I knew I had to do it on my own. Fortunately for me, my studios were pristine and meticulous. They had been cleaned and disinfected every week from day one, so I knew I had that down. But I was unprepared for everything else that would come with the pandemic. With its onset, I promised myself that if I could not keep people safe, first and foremost, then I would close my doors. I would not put anyone at risk or in harm's way. Most of my clientele had autoimmune diseases, various illnesses, cancers, or elderly loved ones at home, and many were stricken by fear and anxiety. They trusted me and the brand that I had built, and I was not going to disappoint them at a time when they needed me most, even if it meant sacrificing myself to do it. So I did just that. I revamped my studios' protocols and procedures, which included additional cleaning and sanitizing procedures. I was in each studio in the early morning, midday, and late evenings to spray down all of my equipment. It was overwhelming, with three studio locations spread throughout the greater Austin area, but I was determined. The safety of my community and my team was a priority to me.

During the two and a half years that followed, I barely slept, and I could feel my health declining again. The stress was unbearable at times. I did all I could to keep my doors open when I was not physically present in the studios. Small businesses, especially in the fitness industry, took a brutal hit. In the first stage of the pandemic, when my studios had to close for two months, I lost 80 percent of my revenue. I continued to pay my staff in full to alleviate any additional stress in their lives. As far as I could tell, no one else was doing this in my industry, but I wanted my team to feel secure when everything else felt insecure. I had built my business from a deep desire, purpose, and passion to help people, and I needed to continue doing that despite losing so much. I was now having to look at ways to cut costs without compromising the integrity of my business or the experience for my community and team.

The lease was ending for one of my studios. It was my first, and it was beautiful, but it was 3,500 square feet, and that kind of space was no longer needed, given the effects that COVID was having on my business. As difficult as it was, I decided to close that location permanently. My heart sank as I called my landlord and told them I would be moving out on April 30, 2020. I had many incredible clients at this location who had been loyal to me and my business from day one. Some would even drive an hour each way to take classes six days a week, no matter the weather. I loved them like family, and this was news I could not deliver to them without great sadness. I had two other studio locations where these clients could take classes, but this one was my first, and I cherished it. We all did.

Then another miracle happened. The morning of April 30, 2020, as I was making plans to notify my clients, move all of my equipment out of that location, and close its doors for good, a developer from Houston called me. He had heard excellent things about my business while on the golf course with some well-known NFL players who came to my studios every time they were in Austin, and he had been pursuing me for over a year to open a business in one of the buildings he owned. I was not mentally or emotionally ready to answer any calls, but my finger did that thing again. It moved to answer the call. I surrendered to this force of nature once again.

The developer did not say hello; he just asked me one question: "What will it take for you to open up in one of my buildings?"

In disbelief at the timing, I paused for a minute to gather my breath and thoughts. I had successfully negotiated three leases before this one, and I knew what I needed, but I could not imagine him saying yes to any of my terms, as I had never asked for them before. But things were different now. Given my business's new circumstances, I asked for everything I would need to make this work for us both. He quickly said yes and agreed to all my terms without hesitation. There were no negotiations; he just agreed to all of them right then and there. I knew intuitively that I had to do it, so I did. Within two hours, our attorneys had my new lease drawn up, and we both signed before I had a chance to talk myself out of it. This developer was a godsend to me, as he even arranged to store all of my equipment at no cost while my new space was under construction. I saw this for the miracle that it truly was. I had listened to my intuition, and it brought me answers that I could not foresee or even imagine on my own.

The new space would take six months to complete. I planned to open it on October 8, 2020. During the build-out, I began working with my investors again to bring my new brand and vision to life. In mid-August 2020, I was in Connecticut meeting with investors from my private equity days and a dear friend from that time who had since branched out to London. While I was having lunch with him in Greenwich, information came across our news feeds that said my current business partner had just pleaded guilty to tax evasion. My friend and I both paused and took in the news. Knowing I needed a plan in case my partner's 50 percent ownership in my business would be affected, we began to discuss all of my options. The friend I was having lunch with, one of the most brilliant and trusted men I know, was well aware of all that I had already been through with this partnership. He also knew of my intense work ethic, and he helped me every step of the way. I also consulted with many other people I knew and trusted, including my legal advisory team. It would take another 18 excruciating, exhausting, expensive, and beyond-stressful months to accomplish, but I was determined. Ultimately, I relinquished a seven-year partnership, took on a new partnership, and saved my business once again. My mission was clear to me. So was my purpose and my passion. But by now, almost nine years in, it felt more like I was constantly rising from my own ashes. Love was no longer the driving force; instead, my mind was driving me, overshadowing my heart and soul and allowing my ego to lead.

While all this was happening, I was losing so much time with my family and so much of myself in the *doing* and not the *living*. My father, who gave me my strength through it all, was now losing his long battle with cancer. My mother was losing her strength as well, and her once-vibrant spirit was breaking more and more with each day. They had been married for 68 years and now their beautiful love story was coming to a painful end.

For me, this was the the culmination of years and years of heartbreak. As the year 2022 began, I had some glimmers of hope, but by February, I finally allowed myself to fall apart. I was breaking, I was broken, and I was done. I did not have the strength to continue in this way. I knew I could no longer allow my thoughts to overpower or confuse me. I also knew that I had to let my intuition guide me. I surrendered wholeheartedly, body and soul.

That was when something happened that I was not expecting. I received a call from a friend who said he knew some investors in

Austin interested in buying my brand—all of it: the name and the company. I knew it was time to move on from this endeavor. I felt it with every ounce of my being. I had built an award-winning brand that I was incredibly proud of, but I knew it was time to let it go. As much as I loved what I had built, it limited me. It was not what I had initially set out to create, and it was at the center of so many painful things that I had experienced to that point. So I said I was interested in speaking to the investors. I gave them a nonnegotiable price. It was well below what it was worth and what I had invested in it, but I needed to move on, so I made it simple. They, of course, accepted my terms and I sold my business within two months. I just wanted to move on and close that chapter of my life and so many others, which I set out to do.

I stayed on for an additional six months to help with the transition. Then I walked away from that business for the last time on November 9, 2022, after almost a decade of undying dedication, innovation, and perseverance. As I drove home that afternoon, I could feel my nervous system, which had kept me in a constant state of fight-or-flight for the past decade, was changing and beginning to relax. My body was finally able to exhale, and my mind could rest. The inner critic that kept me going, even when I knew intuitively that I should not, was finally silenced, and that beautiful sense of serenity, that undeniable trust, calm, and peacefulness that came over me all at once, was confirmation that I had intuitively made the right decision. This was when miracles began to unfold for me, and at a rapid pace, as soon as I arrived home. I will share more about that in the chapters to come *(smiling)*.

The War Within: Mindset versus Intuition

Let's look at what this story reveals about our mindset, aka ego (our deceptive mind), versus gut feeling, first instinct—our intuition. Our truth.

When your mindset and ego move at a velocity much greater than all common sense, they have won the war over your life.

Together, they overpower your intuition with a force beyond recognition. The noise they create derails you and talks you out of your initial gut feeling. Your intuition. Your truth. Feelings of fear, unhappiness, uneasiness, anger, resentment, and hopelessness set in almost immediately. Your mind begins to justify your actions with self-doubt and excuses, and you slip back into your comfort zone, only this kind of comfort is a false sense of security. Like your mindset, it, too, is manufactured. People tend to trust this place because it appears easier. It feels safe because it is known. Yet it is the place of stagnation from which all of your unhappiness stems—the war within.

Your intuition. Your truth. Your saving grace. As unknown and uncertain as these feelings, gut, and instinct may seem to you, they are what will shift your reality into a life fulfilled. Your intuition is the key to so many beautiful things that await you. As fearful as you might be of it now, perhaps always have been, I assure you, it is the doorway to your dreams coming true. Every time I went against my intuition, challenges followed. The challenges became mightier as the themes in my life reoccurred. I kept pushing forward through it all, and in my mind, I believed all of this would bring me happiness one day. In my heart and soul, I intuitively knew differently. But I only trusted my intuition once I was forced to. Looking at all the events that have unfolded in my life, I can clearly see what not trusting my intuition did to me and for me. My intuition always proved accurate. If only I had listened first and foremost. I do now. I allow my intuition to guide me, and my life has been forever transformed in so many beautiful ways because of it. Yours will be, too.

Shedding Your Armor

Our mind is a powerful shield. It builds these walls, this armor. It creates a false sense of security. You must shed this armor that you have put on because you must *feel* your way through this. Your intuition comes through your heart and your soul. It is a sense that can only be felt, and it is a feeling that is undeniable once you open yourself up to it. It is a knowingness that you will not be able to deny once you connect with it. It is your truth, powerful beyond measure. These walls are not protecting you. They are holding you back. Take a deep breath, exhale, and bring them down.

As you bring these walls down, calm will come. Peace of mind will come. Trust will come. Allow the calm to embrace you, the peace of mind to breathe through you, and the trust to enrapture you. Release any and all fear. As we move through this book, this will become clearer to you. The more you let go, the more you will know.

Trusting Your Guidance

Allow your guard to fall and your intuition to guide you now. Trust that it will. It will not fail you. It will not hurt you. It will not lie to you. It will lead you through your transformation in all areas of your life, as you will see. This is where you learn to trust yourself beyond a reasonable doubt, and beyond anything or anyone else. Your intuition will never deceive you; only your mind will.

Flowing and Glowing

When you feel this universal energy align within you, mind, heart, soul, and body, your entire world will light up, as will your body. You will feel the light emanate throughout your entire being brilliantly and beautifully. You will feel the flow of your life as it all comes together and things begin to fall into place for you. You will see challenges as they arise with new eyes, as fear will no longer drive you. You will feel protected, unafraid, and no longer alone, as you will walk in a new way that is in alignment with who you truly are. This is where the magic that is your life begins.

I can say all this with absolute certainty because it happened to me. My transformation came on quickly, and so will yours as you follow along with each chapter of this book.

Your Intuition

*As you work through your mindset and bring your walls down,
are you becoming more aware of your intuitive guidance?*

*Can you recall times in your life when you experienced gut
feelings, first instincts, or intuitive guidance that you followed
and it all unfolded beautifully for you and in ways that
might have even exceeded your expectations?*

*Can you recall times when you experienced gut feelings,
first instincts, or intuitive guidance that you did not follow and
it all unfolded in disaster or disappointment? Looking back at those
experiences, were your initial reactions correct? Were these experiences
recurring themes in your life where lessons needed to be learned?
Were the lessons learned? Did they repeat themselves, with
greater strength each time, until they were learned?*

*Once you define these experiences in your life,
you will be able to see the fear that was the foundation
for all of it. Trust your inner guidance and all fear
will leave your body, not just for now, but forever.*

Note to self: I told you so.

With love, Your Intuition.

Chapter Five

ACCEPTANCE

It Begins with You

The greatest magnifying glasses in the world are a
man's own eyes when they look upon his own person.

— ALEXANDER POPE

I have always found the theory of acceptance intriguing, as it can be perceived in many different ways. Like everything in life, it can work for or against you.

By accepting what was, what is, and what might be, we open ourselves up to change, infinite possibilities, or continued stagnation. It is our choice. We can accept where we are in our lives and believe that is all that there is for us—the limiting belief behind acceptance. Or we can open ourselves up to the infinite possibilities that acceptance will bring to us and our lives if we choose to believe in its limitless essence. It is our choice in how we perceive it and allow it into our lives. Whichever way we utilize it, it is an essential element of healing.

Acceptance is not an invitation to continue to live within the stagnation and restraints of your past or current circumstances, but rather an invitation for you to heal and move past them.

One of the most significant elements of healing is acceptance. Acceptance, for me, meant granting myself peace within for what once had been, what was happening to my body and my life in the present, and what might become of my life, even as unknown as it was to me then. When I finally arrived at this place, after years of resisting, refuting, and suppressing it with all my might, I profoundly found even more peace in my life.

How Acceptance Accelerated My Healing

As I began to devote time to my mindset and overcoming the limiting beliefs that were keeping me bound to mere existence, the moment of clarity that I had hoped for, but did not reasonably believe would ever happen, happened. The moment came on suddenly and unexpectedly. I began to feel this warm light emanating from my body. It was radiant and warm, and it was brilliant. An epiphany came over me that brought with it immense clarity and enlightenment that I felt throughout every ounce of my being. In essence, it was soulful. My deepest fears were dissolved within those moments and have not returned. You will begin to see that the body speaks to you in illness and enlightenment, too.

My entire perception of past events that I had been holding on to so tightly was illuminated right before me in ways that I had not chosen to see—or, shall I say, that I had silenced and decided not to see—my limiting beliefs. Within what felt like mere seconds, so many revelations revealed themselves to me. I allowed myself to become utterly vulnerable to each revelation, as I was finally beginning to understand their true meaning in my life, unlike any of the self-critical definitions I had placed on them before.

It resulted in a massive release from my body that I secretly and knowingly needed with absolute certainty. As I allowed myself to feel each emotion that came through me physically and every feeling I had ever suppressed that I had hidden from everyone—myself included—tears flooded my eyes as if my soul was finally letting go. I allowed these emotions to come through me so that they could finally unburden my mind, body, heart, and soul. I was overwhelmed by the feelings that overflowed through me. First I was submerged in sorrow, loss, grief, regret, and heartbreak. Then the more I accepted all that had occurred in my life to that point with an open heart, the more I released without any excuse or any explanation, the more at peace I became. I was becoming whole again and reconnecting with the deepest parts of my soul, a friendly feeling that I had not felt in a very long time. This is one of the many beautiful benefits of acceptance—the release.

One of the more profound revelations that came to me was the avoidance of my truth, which was born from a deep-rooted *fear* that drove me my entire life. At that moment, I realized fear itself could not be substantiated. It is something that we create and have the ability within us to uncreate. I had to accept that this was all of my own making. I could trace it back to when and where it began in my life, at the young and impressionable age of nine.

Throughout my life, I have moved at an accelerated velocity. I was always building, creating, expanding, educating, learning, researching, analyzing (ad nauseam), designing, engineering, and envisioning all that I had ever hoped to bring to life while pushing through the many obstacles that came my way. They were always coming, and I was constantly overcoming them. I was always hands-on in every aspect of my life. I never stopped to appreciate my accomplishments. I never asked for help or relied on anyone to complete a task with the same care, loyalty, dedication, and precision that I could. I was a perfectionist to a fault. I was never defined by or reliant on my relationships, the men in my life, or my business partnerships. It was always all me, paving my own pathway for the highest good of them all. I seldom slowed down; if I did, it was only during the worst stages of my illness, when I needed to. Even then, I would still find a way to do what needed to get done from home to achieve and reach my goals for my family, my business, and those I wished to help. It never even occurred to me what my choices and levels of stress were doing to my body, which, of course, resulted in the illness that was my wake-up call—waking me up to the phenomenon that our health is not only physical, but mental, emotional, and spiritual. I then had to accept all the choices I had made that worked for me and against me that brought me to this place, and I had to forgive myself for avoiding this truth and not listening to it much sooner, as I could no longer carry on this way.

If you are a perfectionist like I was, you will soon realize that trying to achieve perfection in anything is an illusion, as we are constantly learning and evolving, which means perfection indeed does not exist for any of us. It limits us. We become bound by it. Accepting that unchained me from my restraints. In continually trying to achieve perfection, I felt isolated and utterly alone in my thoughts, which always manifested negatively. I was unavailable to any other possibilities that existed for me to create real change in my life and the lives of so many others. I brought this on myself by believing that I had to do everything on my own. At the moment of realization, I needed to accept this truth and reframe the constructs of my life, and I did. You will too.

The Power of Acceptance and Your Mind

Had I known from the beginning how to silence my inner critic that consistently opposed my intuition, my truth, I would have arrived at this place much sooner, and I could have avoided so many difficult situations. Had I had then the tools I have now, I would have learned these valuable lessons the first time versus having them repeat themselves over and over until I did. The life lessons I denied myself the first time became increasingly painful as I continued on without stopping to get to the root cause of each of them, and without the ability to accept them and then change course. I was not one to blame anyone or anything outside of myself, which left a lot of room for self-blame and self-loathing; I was exceptional at this, but it only made me feel worse and even more alone. For me, acceptance meant knowing and owning the root cause of my pain and no longer creating some excuse or explanation that would make it easy for me to deny my truth. Once I accepted that reality, I had to forgive myself for the time it took to arrive at this challenging conclusion. The decades I had lost then dissolved into hope. By accepting these facts about myself, I could amend these character flaws and release them from my life. Once I did, my mind could no longer use them against me.

Acceptance and Healing

Healing is not linear, nor is there a single path. It is different for every one of us. Our willingness to do the work that brings us back to who we are as souls unites us. Acceptance is an essential element of this journey. Once I understood and accepted what was happening in my life and why, it healed those parts of me that were flawed by unworthiness. It was the only way through it for me. Without acceptance, illness, unhappiness, loneliness, and pain would have limited my inspiration to seek a way forward.

We all wish we could change the past somehow, even though we know we cannot. We also inherently know that no matter how much we try to avoid, suppress, or deny our feelings, we will arrive at the place where we can no longer do this, and that is when we are ready to do our most meaningful work.

You cannot change your past or continue to live within its confinements, so accepting this is essential. Accepting where you are now, without criticizing or condemning your shortcomings and imperfections, will help you rise above them with compassion and grace for where you have been and who you are becoming and will become as a result. You are not who you once were as you are evolving into the highest rendition of yourself.

Accepting your past for what it was, and the lessons learned, forgiving yourself for it, and releasing it from your body will be liberating in its own right. It will take you doing this inner work to experience everything you have not already accepted about your life, current situation, or condition. It was one of the most challenging stages in my healing as I had to take an earnest, honest, and merciless look at how my choices brought me to this place, resulting in multiple illnesses. What I was not seeing or choosing not to see about my life and situation was the big question I asked myself. I had to begin to take responsibility for denying myself what I knew to be true for me and for as long as I did. I know you know what I mean by this. Deep down within you, you know your truth. Accept your truth and surrender to it as I know you can *(smiling)*.

Before this epiphany, I had accepted a mere existence over engaging in life—the acceptance of limiting beliefs. I was comfortably numbed by it all, lifeless in my own body, and in complete disagreement with my very own intuition that would have led me in a very different direction had I chosen to listen to it rather than suppress it time and time again. Once I acknowledged this about my life, it released me from its restraints.

When you accept this element as an essential part of your healing journey, you will realize that no one else can do this work for you but you. Coming to terms with your reality is acceptance in its purest form, and it is yours to surrender to. The transformation you desire is yours to be enraptured by as you persevere through its perfectly timed pirouettes and reflections. You deserve the life you long for, and you will have it. In accepting where you are now, what brought you to this moment in time, and what you will need to do to create the life that you truly desire deep within you, you will begin to see with even more clarity the pathway that you are already paving. The doors will open for you. No climbing into windows is necessary *(smiling)*.

Your deepest desires that you know within your heart and soul to be true for you but have not been willing to speak of, not to yourself or to those closest to you, will be brought to fruition through you. You will begin to explore the depths of your being, all that speaks to you, and the changes in your life that you know you need to make but have been too afraid to until now.

This naturally intrinsic and integral element of your journey begins with you. Only you. You will soon discover what was once undiscoverable to you as you embark upon this essential passageway of your journey toward whole-body healing, forgiveness, and your soul's energy force. Trusting in the process and accepting all aspects of your journey will guide you to your desired destination with courage.

Your Acceptance

As you think about your life, present and past, can you see all the areas you might be holding on to without accepting them for the lessons they came into your life to teach you? Have they held you back in your life? Have you accepted that these experiences make up who you are and that nothing good can come from them? This would be the limiting beliefs of acceptance. Let's flush these out, as they do not support you. Let's write them down, accept them as lessons learned, release them from your mind, heart, soul, and body, and move on from them.

Can you accept what was once unacceptable and forgive what you once believed was unforgivable about these experiences?

Can you see the beauty in them and the strength you gained from them?

Can you accept that they are now in your past and will not interfere with your future?

Can you accept that the person you are today will not be the person you are tomorrow?

With each passing day, you become the person you were meant to become, and all these experiences mold you into this person; in this way, they are incredibly valuable, as are you.

Release your past and accept it for what it was and what it has taught you.

You have the **courage** *within you.*

Chapter Six

COURAGE
Fearlessly Facing Yourself

Valor is stability, not of legs and arms, but of courage and the soul.
— MICHEL DE MONTAIGNE

After you master acceptance for all that once was and now is in your life, you will understand the need for courage to face all yet to come, as stagnation will no longer support you or your journey. You are becoming more and more aware of your surroundings now and becoming conscious of all that has yet to unfold in your life as you move through it. The magic will begin to unfold for you if it hasn't already *(smiling)*. You will understand that courage is not something some of us have; it is something we all have. You are beginning to live consciously.

Living consciously is living courageously.

This means living an authentic, meaningful, and purposeful life bravely. It is not for some of us. It is for all of us. We were all born with a purpose, and the courage and the strength to see it through—including you *(smiling)*. Sometimes it takes immense pain, difficult challenges, or an enduring illness for you to arrive where you are now, ready and willing to be brave and bold and act accordingly, courageously.

When we arrive at this place in our lives, whether forced by our own preconceived limitations or compelled to rise to the occasion, we are exhausted by living in the shadows of our lives. We know, deep within us, that we must move on with our lives even when we do not yet know how. Wherever you are in your journey, you have the courage within you and are ready to embrace your journey now and in a new way.

As you commit to implementing these practices, you will recognize, through clarity, understanding, and acceptance, how you have been hiding behind a facade built by fear all this time. Fear of the truth. Fear of change. Fear of letting go of all that no longer supports your journey toward purpose, fulfillment, and ultimately joy, happiness, health, wellness, peace, and abundance. Shattering these barriers is not only necessary but life-altering, as once you do, your life will come alive in unimaginable and meaningful ways. You will see and experience the beauty of life, miracles in the making in everything you do, and a pathway that unfolds before you that perhaps you would not have allowed yourself to be open to before now.

As you submerse yourself in this work and find clarity within your soul, you will start to see all the things that need to change. As frightening as this might seem to you at this moment, you have what it takes to see it through, and you will. Staying stagnant or remaining paralyzed by fear will no longer be a viable option for you. As afraid as you might be of change, I know that you are more fearful of what your life will become if you stay as you are and where you are now. Staying stagnant will take its toll on you, if it has not already, on your mental, emotional, spiritual, and physical bodies. Taking an honest look at your life is where you need to begin. Find the source or sources of your unhappiness. Evaluate each area of your life, from your relationships to your career, home environment, spirituality, where you live, and with whom you spend most of your time. What brings you joy? What does not? When you answer these two questions in each area of your life, you will understand where your focus must be to create real meaning. And yes, it means fearlessly and courageously facing all that does not bring you joy without hesitation or further avoidance. This is living consciously, aware of all that embodies your life: the good and the not-so-good.

Facing Your Fears

I am sure that your list will not surprise you. Most of the things you need to change most about your life are things you are well aware of because they have been unsettling for quite some time now. We put these things off for as long as possible because they are too intimidating and outside our comfort zone. Well, I am here to tell you, with certainty, you are not comfortable within the restraints of your comfort zone. No one ever is. You think it is your safe place, but it offers no safety. It cannot protect you. It can only delay your healing and your happiness. An authentic and fulfilling life cannot exist within your comfort zone. If you genuinely think about it, it offers no absolute comfort. It is an illusion created by fear.

The gentlest way to put this is: fear is not your friend in illness or health. Fear kept me in a place of stagnation for far too long. Every day that passed, it took more and more away from me. I was miserable living under its power. As unready as I was to face all I knew I needed to, I finally did face it, and it changed everything for me. Instead of living in the shadows of who I once was, I took bold moves in the direction I had always envisioned for my life, toward what I truly wished for and desired. I dove into the depths of the great unknown, releasing all the fear that had once convinced me to stay bound.

Soon after my father passed away, I sold my business. Finally, I walked away from all that I had worked so hard to create, which was, in essence, tying me to a life that I knew was limiting to me and far from what I had set out to achieve in the first place. Knowing that I never fully grieved the loss of my father and the heartbreak that 2022 had brought me, I knew I needed some time to grieve and heal in every area of my life.

The Universe instantly greeted me in a way that had left me no room for doubt. It was as if I let go and the Universe caught me just in time. It was divinely timed, and I was now experiencing it for the first time. Everything began to open up for me in new and magical ways. Ways I was not expecting. The Universe was now supporting me in ways I could physically see and feel deep within my soul.

I knew it when I locked the door to one of my studios for the last time. I did not even need to visit my other two locations for a last good-bye. I knew I was moving on to something more significant in my life. I drove home in a very peaceful state of mind, which was new and refreshing in itself *(smiling)*. I was genuinely unafraid of the future. This feeling of absolute peace was very foreign to me, but I did not question it. I just knew. It was as if my life over the last decade was already a distant memory and I had already moved on from it.

It took every ounce of courage I could muster up to finally let go of that life I had created for myself that I had held on to for as long as I did, even through the most tragic events. But I did it, and you can too. It released me, and I did not realize how much I needed the release. It was unbelievably freeing. It bestowed upon me a new-found sense of hope and faith that I could not honestly explain, as up to this moment I had lost both faith and hope.

I returned home and went straight into my bedroom and lay down. Valletta and Luc were still at school, so I had some time to relax into these feelings that were so new and all-consuming for me. I utterly and wholeheartedly surrendered to the next chapter in my life, whatever that might be. I felt the fears I had been holding on to for over a decade slip away from my body.

Then my mobile phone started vibrating as I was lying there, embracing the silence and the peacefulness of it all. I did not wish to be bothered but was compelled to have a look. That is when I noticed a text from my friend, author Elizabeth Hamilton Guarino. We had not spoken in over 11 years because our lives had been so busy, but I felt compelled to read her text. She was asking me if I had some time for a call to catch up that evening. I didn't want to speak to anyone yet, but my fingers repeated that soulful step that the Universe divinely orchestrated once again. My fingers moved to respond. *Yes, let's speak this evening. I will be available after 8 P.M.* Send. It is what my soul moved me to write through my body without any involvement from me. I could not believe I had just committed to catching up with an old friend on the same day all this was happening, but I knew I needed to do it. Looking back, I can see how I was closing one chapter and opening a new one—a beautiful future aligned with who I am and my soul's purpose. Within minutes of walking away from my former life, I went from living with a chronic fear of the future to fearlessly allowing something much greater than me to lead me. For someone like me, that was unimaginable, yet I could not question any of it. I just knew, with every ounce of my being, that I had made the right choice and was now on the right path because of it. Something I had dreaded doing for years was finally done, and the Universe was now supporting me fully.

After my children came home from school, we had dinner, and I shared the news with them. My children, who had grown up accustomed to me working 24/7/365, were utterly shocked. They never thought I would ever walk away from my business, as it was my heart and soul in many ways. I was helping people live healthier lives, which was my passion, and I did it on a grand scale. As a family, we discussed what was next for me and for us. Not only was I selling the business that I had built that took me away from them for much of their upbringing, but we were also going to move out of the country. This was something I had always wanted to do. I had attempted it twice and was always swayed away from it by men I had fallen in love with *(smiling)*. I was set to move for the second time when I met and married Mitch. The timing was not right then, but I made him promise me that we would move our family to Europe within 10 years of our marriage. That hadn't happened on the 10-year timeline, but now it was time, and no one would stop me. I was no longer afraid to make a move for fear of losing someone, because I had learned that in doing so, I lost myself. Another fear I needed to face, and I did.

My family's lineage originated in the Crown Colony of the Island of Malta and its Dependencies, confirmed under the Treaty of Paris in 1813, which formalized the transfer of power from France to Britain. So, being a French-British Maltese (an island girl at heart) with an undeniable loyalty to British-made vehicles and all things French, my destination for my family has always been my most beloved city: Paris, France, a train ride away from London and a direct flight to the south of France. We could make this happen with our dual citizenship, and it was now time. My children's task was to finish the school year and learn French while we prepared for the most significant move of our lives. As scary as this could have been, I was unafraid, as I was now in a brave pursuit to fearlessly face every hope, dream, and destination my heart desired. After all, I had worked hard my entire life, and for the first time, this was about me. My future was unknown to me, and I believed the pathway to my family moving to Paris had finally opened for me.

The Courage That Comes with Trusting the Process

Then something miraculous and magical happened again, followed by many supernatural events. Elizabeth called me as I was cleaning up the kitchen after supper and mindfully settling into my new life. I was still enjoying a sense of peace that had not yet left me, and to this day still has not. We spent the first hour of our call catching up on our lives and our families. Then Elizabeth told me that I should write a book about everything I had been through to get to this place. Elizabeth is a fantastic woman with lots of energy and charisma; when she says something, action follows close behind. I had always known I would write a book one day, and it felt like the right time. Elizabeth did not hesitate; she said she would introduce me to her agent, who happened to be one of the best in the industry, based out of New York City. Every ounce of my body lit up with a light that emanated within me and radiated brilliantly. It was a deepening of the feelings I had been experiencing all afternoon.

After our call ended, I just sat with it for a while. I knew something was guiding me, and I trusted it. I would not force anything, but allow it to unfold as I intuitively knew and trusted it would. This was me releasing all fear from my body, something I never thought I could do, but I had this newfound courage that came with trusting the process that was now leading me.

The following day, I woke up and checked my e-mail. To my surprise, I had a message from a friend, the executive vice president of a major fitness manufacturer who had been involved in helping me bring my new brand to life pre-COVID. COVID had halted those plans for me, but now my friend was e-mailing me to see where I was at with my new brand. Before I could stop to think, my fingers did that thing again. Without hesitation, I hit reply and started writing. Words were flowing through me as if something else was writing it for me before I could have the opportunity to talk myself out of it—something I might have done before now. At a rapid speed, my fingers typed that I would get back to him with the new design of my new machine within a few weeks and wished him a happy Thanksgiving. Then I hit send, all the while observing my body act independently without me getting in the way. It was November 10, 2022, not even 24 hours after I had left my former business model behind me. I sat there at my desk and took it all in once again. It had been almost two years since he and I last spoke, and I now saw this as another sign that something much more significant than me was guiding this.

I intuitively knew I needed to redesign my machine, as I no longer wanted to use my original CAD (computer-aided design) plans.

I also knew I needed a new engineer to produce the CAD drawings for my redesigned machine, as it had to be unique to my new vision and concept, which had changed over the years. As the day went on, I realized that something profound was happening in my life and it was not time to rest my body just yet. I spent most of that day researching engineers, as I wanted a specific type of person to bring this to life in a way that my original machine had not been. I created a list of two dozen different engineers from all over the world. I e-mailed each of them about what I needed to bring my creation to life without giving away the details. I then said to myself that I would not force this. It would happen naturally, without issue or hesitation, if it were to happen. I was allowing the Universe to continue to lead me. I told myself that the first engineer to respond would be the one whom I would work with.

At 2 A.M., I was lying in bed thinking about the last 24 hours. Not about the business I had left, but about what had happened since letting it go. The fear I had naturally felt in every part of my day was gone. I had faced so many of my fears in this last year that I could now see my life changing, and quickly, too. I was in my element and on my intended path, and I was no longer fighting it from fear.

As I contemplated the events unfolding, an e-mail came in from an engineer from a faraway country. From what I could tell by my feelings about our communication, he was young, eager, and brilliant. He was very polite and well mannered. I admired this about him. He signed my very long and detailed new mutual NDA that I had had my attorney draft for me earlier that day, and then we spent the next few hours going back and forth over text.

I am not a big fan of this type of communication, but it was late, and I was not about to get the camera ready for a Zoom call with anyone (LOL). I explained to the young engineer in great detail what I was looking to create. He then said, and I quote, *I will bring your dream to life for you. I will send it to you by Thanksgiving Day.* That was exactly two weeks away. He did not know that that was the date I had promised my friend I would get the new CAD designs to him. I had complete faith that this was my engineer and that the timing would be in sync with the promise my fingers put into writing without my human involvement (LOL).

I could now physically see and feel the tangible effects of clearing my mind from the noise, following my intuition, accepting all that had happened in my life and was happening now, and courageously and fearlessly following through for the first time without hesitation. It was all becoming so clear to me, and it was all manifesting so profoundly and in ways that I could not have created nor even imagined. It all began when I followed my first gut instinct to sell my business when investors approached me and did not allow my mind to overturn that decision, which my inner critic tried many times to do *(smiling)*. I am sharing this part of my story with you so you can see how quickly your life will transform when doing this work, as I know it will.

The very next day, I woke up to a text from Elizabeth letting me know that her agent was open to a call with me and that she would introduce us via e-mail. The e-mail was already in my inbox, and her agent had already responded. Elizabeth was one to make things happen, as I was, so I knew that when she said she would do something, she would follow through. We then set up a call to speak. I was in awe. I had always felt I would write a book someday—several, to be exact—and now it was being realized. Always in the past I would talk myself out of it, but not this time, as I no longer allowed those thoughts in. I was in control of them by this time. They no longer existed for me—and still do not.

I trusted the process for the first time in my life. I was in the natural flow of events unfolding, moving through and with the flow of it all. The synergy felt natural to me, and I knew the Universe was guiding me, so I trusted in that for the first time in my life. I was genuinely unafraid of what the future before me held. I was so excited by it all. I had not felt that in a long time, and it felt fabulous! You will see *(smiling)*.

The next day, the agent and I had our call. He was very much a New Yorker, which I loved. Very direct and straight to the point. I admire those qualities in a person very much. He told me that I would need to write a book proposal, and he then told me how difficult it was to get published as a first-time author. He was honest and open about the process and what I could expect, not knowing I had no expectations. I trusted the magic of it all and knew it would unfold how it was meant to or destined for me. I left it in the hands of the Universe, something I had not done before. As we ended our call, he said he would e-mail a book proposal guideline for me to see so I could understand the process. Then he said he would read over my book proposal when it was ready and let me know his thoughts. He did not commit to signing me, representing me, or distributing my book proposal at this point. I admired his honesty and valued his time.

With the holidays approaching and our family spending them without my father's presence for the first time, I knew it would be difficult for all of us. So I told the agent I would have a proposal to him by early 2023. I had never written a book proposal before but knew intuitively I could. I loved writing, and this was the next step toward this part of my journey.

As the days went by leading up to Thanksgiving, I was thinking about everything that had happened that year and spending some time healing from it all. I then took some time to watch a series that was streaming on my iPad. I searched for a good-quality series that could take my mind off everything and allow me to lose myself in it for just a few hours. While I was searching the shows, a name I knew came across the screen—something I had not noticed before but knew I was meant to now. It was Lorenzo Agius, my cousin from London. Lorenzo had become one of the world's most sought-after celebrity photographers. He and his brother Alfie Agius (who had played in the rock band The Fixx) lived in London with their families. My mother, who was with me during this time, had been communicating with our family overseas since my father's passing, so I thought it was time I did too.

I contacted Lorenzo that evening, and we had a wonderful conversation. I was set to travel back to Paris in January, so we arranged to see one another in London while I was there in Europe. I knew that if I was going to embark on this new journey, I needed to be represented well and captured with all my heart and soul, and Lorenzo was the photographer who could capture just that in the people he photographed. This man has more heart and soul than anyone I have ever met; his work is a grand representation of his heart and soul. His work is art in its most brilliant and beautiful form. I had not worked with him yet, but I knew it was time. It was yet another piece that was magically falling into place. The Universe was putting all the pieces together for me, and it will do the same for you too.

I was beginning to observe that my inner critic no longer had any hold over me and that my intuition was divinely leading me, connecting me to a source deep within me, openly guiding me. I was following it without any doubts or delays, and I was beginning to see the results of the work I had done that brought me to this place. These results came quickly with my epiphany. It was, in itself, a beautiful and welcoming miracle unfolding right before me. All I had to do now was to follow through courageously and without fear. I was committed. These events could not be explained or analyzed. They had to be experienced, and I was experiencing them.

Fast-forward to Thanksgiving morning. I woke up to an e-mail from my engineer. I took a deep breath and opened it up, and one by one, I saw 44 CAD designs of my new machine that brought me to my knees with gratitude and tears of absolute joy. I was illuminated as I looked at each design. Tears ran down my face as I realized my pathway was unfolding before me and through me. I had to let go, trust, and flow with the energy even more. It was yet another sign along this journey of enlightenment and transformation.

This man whom the Universe brought to me in the middle of the night did bring my dream to life as he said he would and as I trusted that he would. It was as if he could see this machine I had been designing in my mind for the past eight years in a way the engineers before him could not grasp. I was so excited that my body did that thing again where I moved in ways I was not in control of (LOL). I clicked on Forward and sent the e-mail to my friend, who had requested it two weeks prior. I wished him and his family a happy Thanksgiving and told him he could get back to me after the holidays. Just a few minutes later, he wrote me right back, letting me know that this machine was aesthetically and mechanically the most beautiful machine he had ever seen. He then asked my permission to send it on to his four leading manufacturers in China and Taiwan. These were four of the top five manufacturers in the world, so of course I said yes, provided that they would all sign my mutual NDA, which they did. Within 24 hours, they all got back to him individually. They all loved the machine and would be bidding on it to be my manufacturer. Before I could decide, I was introduced to the fifth manufacturer in the top five, from Italy, by a mutual friend whom I had always trusted and was also very interested. Over the next few months and into the new year, I discussed my machine with all five of my dream manufacturers. It was surreal, as it is so difficult to get one manufacturer on board and interested, let alone five. It was another miracle, another confirmation that I was on the right path and my dreams were unfolding in ways that exceeded my imagination.

I was entering the new year and traveling between London and Paris, meeting with investors, former colleagues, and dear friends I had always respected, admired, and adored. It was so wonderful to be back in these two cities. While traveling to London to meet with Lorenzo and a former colleague, I was beginning to think more about my book and proposal. I was halfway through it and taking this time abroad to pull it all together; it had always been within me, but now it was being brought to life. I could see how my life got me to where I could honestly do the work I always knew I needed to. I was amazed by everything happening in my life and how quickly it had all changed for me once I did.

As I wrapped up my travels and headed back to the States, I used my time on the flight home to work more on my book proposal. As I landed and turned my airplane mode off, my mobile flooded with e-mails and texts. The first one I saw was from my soon-to-be agent *(smiling)*. It was very simple, straight to the point and in perfect timing, asking me when I would have my book proposal to him. This was late in the evening on Saturday, February 11, and I quickly wrote back: *In the way of the divine (smiling), I will have it to you by Valentine's Day.* My body just moved to write that date, and I did not question it. It was one of my favorite days of the year, so I thought it was appropriate. As promised, I worked on my book proposal for the next two days and then sent it to him on Valentine's Day. I had requested that he send it to Hay House before any others. I loved Louise Hay, whose book *You Can Heal Your Life* changed the trajectory of my life in my early 20s, and I always knew that when I wrote my first book, I wanted to be published by Hay House. It was a dream of mine to work with them, as I felt they were helping people in profound ways and I wanted to be a part of it.

So my agent sent my proposal off to Hay House. Within weeks, my publishing deal was done. I was absolutely amazed by it all—divinely guided and perfectly timed. *Miracles in the making.*

When I left my business for the last time, I had planned to take time off, continue healing and grieving, get my family ready to move, and figure out the next chapter of my life. The Universe had different plans for me. As I began doing this work, it all began to unfold. It was all happening naturally and rapidly. It will for you too.

By having the courage to face my fears and do this work, I saw everything in my life begin to change. By accepting the offer on my business and following through with the sale, in defiance of my inner critic, I let go of so much that I knew I needed to. Within hours of walking away from it, new pathways began opening up for me, and I knew they were leading me to what I had set out to create initially. I can look back now and see why my illness came about and why my healing took so much longer than it needed to. It was all built on the foundation of fear. I lacked the courage to make these changes until I was forced to. Once I dared to move through it and above it all, the fear melted away, and it no longer exists for me, even to this day.

The magic and miracles are everywhere in my life now, and they will be for you too. With all my heart and soul, I can say this to you, because it happened in my life. This work might feel challenging at first, but that will soon pass, and it will lead you into a life you cannot imagine until you live within it. It is just that beautiful. Beyond beautiful. You have the courage and strength to see this through, and you will—*bravely and boldly.*

Your Courage

*Can you look back upon your life and see
all the experiences you allowed to happen or stayed
in from a place of comfort or fear? Can you see where these
experiences have disappointed you, held you
back, hurt you, and betrayed you?*

*Can you see into them with an open, honest heart,
and can you see what you feared most about these experiences?
Can you see when, deep within you, you knew you had to
create change but did not have the courage to do so?*

*Can you see where finding the courage
that is already within you to make these changes will
lead you to the life that you desire? Can you see how releasing
fear from your life will benefit every area of your life?*

*Can you recall experiences when you had the courage
to follow your heart and it unfolded beautifully? Can you recall what
that felt like for you? What miracles came with it?*

*Can you see how your life will transform by
courageously, fearlessly, and bravely following your heart
and allowing it all to unfold as you work through it?*

*The Universe will open the passageways for you
as you do this work. Commit to your transformation
with courage and without fear, and you will
see it happen with* **grace**.

part III

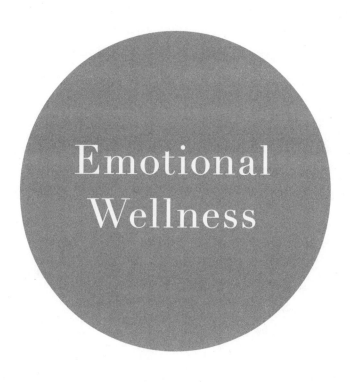

Emotional Wellness

Chapter Seven

GRACE

Loving Yourself

To go back is impossible in existence . . .
It's not about disappearing into the ocean,
but of becoming the ocean.

— KAHLIL GIBRAN

You are now opening up to the infinite possibilities of your life, and there is so much yet for you to experience and discover in all of your beauty, imperfections, and reflections. You are, and have been all this time, transcending who you once were. Your truth is becoming known to you. It is in your truth and in loving yourself that you will see all that awaits you, even in times of trepidation. You have been finding your way through it all to a place where even these times will no longer hinder your future, progress, and recovery. Once you gently reawaken and see everything you have been hiding behind, you will understand why your body needs to slow you down to listen. The answers to all of your questions are already within you. Not outside of yourself. Not in anyone else. Love yourself enough to listen to your body; it will not guide you astray. Allow it to lead you and follow the flow of universal knowledge waiting to bring so many magical, meaningful, and miraculous moments into your life.

Loving Who You Are

Loving who you are is the essence behind this body of work and what it means to love yourself truly. It is not about anything outward that takes you inward. It is about bringing what is within you *out* and becoming boundlessly vulnerable to the knowledge within you that is inviting you on this journey of a lifetime. You will not believe this until you let go and journey forward.

Many people believe that "loving yourself" means taking care of yourself from the outside in, with an overabundance of beauty treatments, massages, and anything and everything you can lavishly leverage to help you feel outwardly loved. Though these things are important in many ways, they are not the foundation of graciously loving yourself for the beautiful body of light that you are. Truly loving yourself begins with grace—for your journey and all it has taught you thus far and where it is now taking you. In loving the good and the not-so-good about who you are and who you once were, you will come to understand how important it is to offer yourself unconditional love in all areas, even in the deepest and darkest depths of your being where you need it the most. Once you do this—truly do this—the darkness will lift, and you will see a way forward that is beautifully lit up just for you. You will evolve into the person you know you are in your very essence, the person you have always wished to become. There is no holding back. No apologies. This is not a selfish act, it is an essential one, and this work will naturally bring this to light as you courageously journey forward.

We are all guilty of diminishing ourselves for the choices of our past, as they still haunt us in many ways. Well, the reality is they do not need to haunt us. They only haunt us in our memories of them and the meanings that we have placed on them. Rather than continuing to live within these memories we have created, we can move on from them completely. It is time for you to do so now. You cannot change any of it. You can only clear a pathway free from these memories and restraints. Learn from them, *accept them*, heal them, and allow yourself to move on from them. We all make mistakes; they bring us to this place where we can see them, learn from them, and never repeat them. If you repeat them, you are only teaching yourself and others that this is all you are worthy of, when you are truly worthy of so much more. But you must be the one to see that first by relinquishing the cycle and learning to love yourself through it all.

People will only see the parts of you that you allow them to see. Now it is time for them to see you for who you are. If you fear people will not accept and love you for who you are, love yourself enough to release them from your life. Family included.

Your Body Is Your Sanctuary

This body you are in is home to your soul, your energy force. You must cherish and protect it above all else, as it is the vessel your soul speaks and moves through. Looking at ourselves with nothing but love for what we see can be difficult, but it should not be. You will learn to love yourself in every facet as you connect more deeply with your inner self.

At various times in our lives, our reflections in the mirror may not always please us. Still, even in those moments, our thoughts do not define us as we sometimes believe that they do, as our reflections continuously evolve as we do. This body is a miraculous creation with endless possibilities and healing abilities. It will follow suit as you support it with love and allow it to do what it naturally can and wants to do for you. Once you align with it, it will heal you from everything you cross paths with—mind, heart, soul, and ultimately, body.

You are not at war with yourself, even when it feels like you are. Once you align your thoughts (unconscious and conscious), your intuition (energy force), and your heart and soul, the courage to persevere will become natural, and you will become unstoppable. In facing yourself, taking that deep dive within your being, and then healing the self-image you set for yourself, you will begin evolving, as you will soon witness. You are more than capable of all of this, and I know that you are at a place in your life where this is essential for you to do now. So step even deeper into this great unknown and let it be known to you, as it will reveal itself to you when you are ready. And you *are* ready.

Your Body Is Your Beacon

In my darkest days, it was easy to blame my body for failing me, and I did at every step. I could easily have continued to blame so many things outside of myself without looking at what I did to my body to cause my illness. I accepted stagnation and allowed circumstances that I knew within me were not meant for me. I internalized and analyzed everything. I lived within the void of my own making, allowing my mind to betray me through the worst events. There were so many interferences and distractions, but the truth is that I allowed them to come into my life and, in turn, caused my body to become unwell. But at the time, I could not see the truth. I was very much in denial and completely shut down. My reality was hidden from me—until I deeply dove into the ocean in which I was drowning. I had to face myself and my way forward, and I did. I stumbled a lot, and you will, too, but then I found solid ground, and you will, too. Give yourself grace and love yourself through it. That love will grow even deeper as you move through this journey.

Love Yourself Enough to Let Go

From my darkest point on, for the next seven years, I vacillated between the truth that I knew and that I denied myself until I found the courage to stay on course. That courage finally came with selling my business.

I can see it so clearly now, looking back. When the mutiny within my business began, I knew it. I physically felt it. I have always been a very empathic and intuitive person in this way. Even at my most shut down, I could feel the energy around me very strongly. I could walk into any of my studios and I would know. I could always feel the energy and understand it without question. Within weeks of the mutiny beginning, I intuitively knew what was happening. At the point where I could not deny it, I called my leading attorney and explained.

Knowing me as he does, my attorney could not understand why anyone I had hired would want to do this to me. But we were dealing with dishonorable people—four in particular who were at the helm of it all. I realized I could have expected this treatment from them, but not from the rest of my team. That was where I felt the most betrayed. My team all knew but did not say anything to me. They betrayed my trust with each passing day.

Six months into this mutiny, I let go of one of the main offenders. Then I let go of seven others who were influenced by that person and involved in trying to control the rest of my team. Once the arbitration was over, I let go of more people involved as the details revealed themselves, and this went on for the next few years. By the time I sold the business, most of the people involved were gone, except for one person I kept on who had moved to Austin to work for me and who had dependents I was concerned about. This was a mistake, and if I had it to do over again, which I do not, I would have let this person go from the moment I recognized I could not trust them. Letting go may seem painful initially, but holding on will become more painful the longer you continue it.

Love yourself enough to make the difficult decisions necessary to keep your peace and the peace of those around you and those you love. *It is all love.*

Protecting Your Energy Is Love

Energy is vital, and protecting yours is central to loving yourself. In selling my business, I learned that I had placed the energy and the needs of others before my own, and this is where I failed myself during this time. I supported my team and community in many ways but did not support my own needs, as I always put everyone else first. But not anymore. I am supporting myself first and foremost now, and you will too. In learning to love myself, put myself first, and protect my own energy, I have come to have complete trust in the Universe to guide me and bring the right people into my life. I have learned to honor myself by loving myself. I am in oneness with who I am and what I need. So, if someone's energy does not feel right to me, I know they are unsuitable for me, and I do not engage with them. In loving yourself, you honor yourself, too. This is not a selfish act; it is a necessary one.

Your Grace

*Where in your life can you give yourself grace for all you have been
through, who you once were, and who you are becoming?*

*Can you love your body knowing it is home to the magic
that awaits you? Can you see beyond the physical
and into the spiritual aspects of your body?*

*Can you unconditionally love every aspect of your being
and body without faltering, knowing that it has not
betrayed you, only lit your pathway home?*

*Can you love yourself enough to let go of the energy,
or energies, that surround you that no longer protect your peace?*

*Can you love yourself enough to protect your energy
and your peace from that which surrounds you?*

*Graciously love yourself and allow your **healing** to begin.*

Chapter Eight

HEALING

It Begins with Forgiveness

Natural forces within us are the true healers of disease.

— HIPPOCRATES

Healing. It is a profoundly powerful word that has many meanings for our existence. Healing is not something we need to do in only one area of our lives; it is something we must do in all areas of our lives to embrace our true selves. Our souls. The light that emanates from within us.

In healing from all you have ever allowed to define you, you must journey back to where it began, that fragile place in time when everything changed for you. When you silenced your spiritual being and ushered in your human being, putting you in a state of discord within yourself, making oneness impossible.

The onset of challenges and the recovery from them are neither the beginning nor the end of your journey toward healing. They are both catalysts for your passage inward toward your light, reminding you of your brilliance, beauty, and brightness. Healing is your mental, emotional, spiritual, and physical way of reawakening. It serves a profound purpose in your life by dismantling it so that you can reconstruct it in a new and powerful way.

Once I realized how powerful this truth was, I did everything I could to heal every part of me that had brought me to this place in my life. Before this epiphany, I did not truly understand that my life leading up to my illness had brought the illness on. My pathway to recovery from illness was my reawakening to my truth.

Embodying Your Truth

Every choice I had ever embodied that was not in alignment with my truth brought me to a place where my physical body had to slow me down because I had circumvented all of the signs along the way—and there were so many. I was solely responsible for making these choices, and now it was time to be accountable for them, heart and soul. My soul was now demanding it. The years leading up to the onset of the physical signs of my illness were the most challenging for me, and the most telling, as I look back upon them. My once vibrant and ambitious life had taken a turn I could not have foreseen. I had lost faith in my intuition. I had stopped believing in it, and I had stopped listening to it. I had silenced it like so many of us do. I went from a conscious and spiritual life to an unconscious one. Fear had taken hold of me, and anxiety became my new comfort zone—a loveless and emotionless place built on the foundation of fear. It was distracting and diverting me from the life I knew I desired to live, the magic that awaited me, and the truth that I had always felt deep within my soul that I could not understand or express at the time but can now *(smiling)*.

By a force of nature much greater than I, I was forced out from within this comfort zone, only realizing several years later how comfortless it truly was. I was never genuinely safe within its barriers, yet I gave it so much power over me. Creating the life I desired seemed impossible. I was too afraid even to try. Fear was at the center of it all, and overcoming my fears and facing the many truths I had been avoiding is when it all began for me and where it will begin for you—healing every part of you.

Healing Beyond the Physical Body

When I began my journey toward healing, I set out to heal my physical body first because that is where my symptoms began to present themselves to me. I did not understand at the time that this was an internal phenomenon that manifested externally, so I focused on the external, what I could physically "see" and "feel." By "feel," I mean the physical symptoms taking over my life, not the emotions and fear I had been suppressing that were at the center of it all. The physical signs of my illness came on very quickly, within seconds, as I shared in earlier chapters. The physical signs were undeniable and very apparent, which is why I started my healing by addressing them with six weeks of acupuncture therapy, but I soon came to realize that this, alone, was not the answer. At the end of my six weeks of treatment, I could feel 90 percent of my facial muscles return, but the 10 percent that I still could not feel sent me into the unknown so that it could be known to me.

The 10 percent of my facial muscles that remained paralyzed, along with the new symptoms that were continuing to present themselves to me with each new day, thrust me into an intense depression that would lead me, four years later, to my very first miracle and lay the foundation for my healing. During the four years that preceded my very first miracle in recovery, I focused only on the symptoms that were slowing me down and bringing my life to a halt, not the underlying reasons why my body had taken these extreme measures to get my attention. Every doctor and specialist I saw over those years said the same thing: my body was attacking itself. I heard this repeatedly, but the doctors and specialists had no concrete explanation for what was happening to me. They did what most do: put me in a one-size-fits-all box and prescribe me anything and everything, the same things they prescribed to everyone else, to try to keep my symptoms at bay. This approach was like a Band-Aid on a wound—and the wound never healed in this way.

One thing that I knew without question, even back then, was that it was not my body attacking itself. I know now that it was me. I was not true to myself and had not been for a long time. I had allowed myself to become a shell of the person I once was, void of the beauty I had once seen in the world and in everything that crossed my path. I found myself in a volatile situation that was not of my own making, facing circumstances that I did not invite into my life. But I had taken a vow and was committed to seeing my husband and our family through it.

This was in 2011, while we still lived in California. Without going into too much detail, we found ourselves threatened by a person causing such drama and chaos for our family that on the advice of a dear friend, FBI profiler and hostage negotiator Clint Van Zandt, we decided to quietly move out of state and head to Texas, where we could offer our family protection that we could not receive in California. Our son, Luc, was only 8 months old; our daughter, Valletta, was 26 months old. We were building our first home together. But we knew that walking away from it was the safest option for our family.

Starting again in Texas was not what I had ever imagined for our life. *My* life. Still, I knew that I could do it and that I had to do it. But the minute that I let my guard down, began to breathe, and decompressed from all that had happened in our lives to bring us to Texas, that was when I woke up to Bell's palsy. Living in a constant state of fight-or-flight for as long as I had activated my sympathetic nervous system in its response, causing my body so much distress and unrest. This happened within six months of our move; it was the beginning of my reawakening, and the first of my wake-up calls, but not the last. The more I focused my healing externally on my symptoms and not the underlying causes, the more unwell I became. This is when my journey into whole-body healing began.

As my body began to respond and heal with food as my medicine, as I described in an earlier chapter, I began to look at the inner conflicts that brought me to this place of illness. I am by nature a very analytical person, so as wonderful as getting my health back was, I needed to look deeper into why this had happened to me in the first place.

I began analyzing every aspect of my life leading up to my illness. Everything surrounding me, from my family to my business, my team, my community, and the current state of my life. Everything and everyone I had ever shared time with before my illness and since. Those feelings deep within me that I had been avoiding and not dealing with. The internal conflicts had manifested into illness. I knew that I was off my path and far from my center. I knew so many changes needed to happen, and I was the only one who could make them happen. I had to follow my truth.

Since I owned my own business and had a family to consider, I had to be strategic in planning the changes that needed to take place for me and my family to live a more meaningful, fulfilling, and purposeful life. Whole-body healing—not just my illness—was now at the center of my thoughts. My focus was on every ounce of my being: my mental health (mindset), my spiritual health (intuition), my emotional health (loving myself), my physical health (strengthening my body), and my overall well-being. I was coming into my own by creating oneness within. I soon came to realize that all these aspects of well-being work together. You cannot have one without the others. This is a beautiful synergy of truths that, once realized, can be actualized into infinite, limitless, and boundless opportunities for growth.

Finding Forgiveness Within

The most challenging aspect for me was my mental wellness, since this meant eradicating the narrative within me that misguided, misled, and prorogated my growth and left my emotional wellness depleted, defeated, and lifeless, so that I was merely existing and not engaging in my life. It meant observing and reframing my thoughts before they dissolved into the lifelessness from which they spawned. It took great courage to see these thoughts for what they were. When I found the courage to face and accept them, my emotional wellness began improving. I could now shine light into the shadows within me and slowly began to release myself from the burdens, limitations, and restraints I had set in motion. Once I was no longer at war with my mindset, my journey toward emotional healing began. It began with forgiveness, grace, and a deeper understanding of what brought me to this place. It was not where my story ended but where my story truly began.

By nature, we are emotional creatures, and when our emotional wellness does not align with our mental wellness, our lives become filled with conflict and confusion—the war within. Our thoughts dictate our behavior in this place, leaving us powerless over them and hopeless before them. You can feel the tension and stress running throughout your body when you are in this place. It leaves you feeling defeated. It is where who you once were and who you are becoming disappear until you are ready to resurface—the space in between these two worlds.

By deepening your understanding of your current state of mind and emotions, you align and restore peace within. This is where forgiveness can be found, healing every element of you that you have kept hidden from the world to see and experience in your purest form. Forgiveness is the hardest thing for us to do when it should be rudimentary in understanding that you cannot change your past and no longer need to be bound by it or to it. When we allow our past, or the people from it, to haunt us, hold us back, and define us and our worthiness, we stay devoted to pain instead of committed to our healing and growth because we can no longer see anything else for ourselves. Holding on to the past keeps us believing that is all we will ever be or become, which is the furthest thing from the truth. Your truth. Forgiving who you once were, the choices you once made in that state of being, and the people who played their roles in it are essential. Forgiveness releases you from the pain you hold on to and gives you the strength to move through it and on from it. Leaving it where it needs to be: in your past. Once you forgive yourself, you can seek forgiveness from those you wish it from.

You Will Be Healed

Healing is something you can do, and I know that you will. It will take your willingness to heal and bring light upon the parts of you that you have kept hidden from all to see, including those closest to you. The emotions that you suppressed, forsook, and abandoned because, at the time, it was so much easier for you to do rather than bring them to the surface to face them, heal them, resolve them, and release them. It is now time for you to do just that, and you will because you know deep within that it is your desire. In your healing journey, all of these emotions that have stayed with you have affected you on a cellular level, whether you are conscious of this or not. If you do not work through these emotions and continue to hold on to them and suppress them, they will manifest in other forms until you do. If they have not already, they will find their way to the surface of your life in ways of anger, irritability, sadness, depression, anxiety, fear, loss, grief, loneliness, and changes in the body (weight gain or weight loss, hair loss) and inevitably, changes in your overall health and wellness. My repressed emotions manifested in a debilitating illness that took me years to discover and recover from.

The Heart of Healing

Healing your mind, soul, and body is essential in living consciously and the life we truly desire and deserve. In healing emotionally, we get to the heart of it all—healing the emotions within us that feel the darkest and heaviest. The places within us that are void of all light and home to the burdens we have chosen to carry for ourselves and others. In healing, we are releasing ourselves of these burdens, thoughts, feelings, and emotions that bring us the most uneasiness, unhappiness, and uncertainty so that we can move forward with confidence and grace toward our soul's purpose with an inner knowingness we can no longer deny ourselves.

Once you reach this place, you will know with absolute certainty as you will feel it within every ounce of your being. Deep within you, you are already well aware of the emotions that you must amend, heal, and move on from, and once you do, your pathway will light up for you. It will reveal to you your soul's purpose. Get ready to light your own way.

Your Healing

Deep within you, you know your truth.
Can you gently bring that to the center of your life now,
heal all the parts of you that kept it hidden from all to see,
and forgive all those involved, including yourself?

Can you feel the feelings within your body that your body
has held on to and dive deep within them to heal them?

Can you now find forgiveness for your war within
and all that brought you to this place?

In doing this work, you will heal in all areas of your life.
Can you believe this for you now?

Can you forgive yourself now?

Understand the process of **trauma** *and overcome*
the pain of the events that have shaped our lives.

Chapter Nine

TRAUMA

Honoring the Pain and Releasing It

The cure for pain is in the pain.

— R U M I

Trauma comes into our lives in many ways and many forms. Through loved ones, family, friends, world events, workplaces, and acquaintances, and sometimes inherited across generations and lifetimes. It is inescapable and a part of life as we know it, but does it have to continue throughout our lives? That is the biggest question I asked myself after the events that changed everything for me. We are all born into this world with lessons we need to learn in this lifetime to evolve in the way we are meant to. Each life lesson is unique and always aligns with our soul's purpose. By now, you might be well aware of the life lessons that you most need to learn in this lifetime. If not, you will soon be made aware of them. You may have been fighting them all of this time, but deep down within you, you know what these life lessons are for you.

The Events That Shape Our Lives

These lessons are in the events that repeatedly play out in our lives. With each event, the players may change, and the circumstances may change, but the lesson is still at the heart of it and is still the same. These life lessons will repeat themselves with greater and greater force behind them until you become conscious of them in such a way that change can finally occur. If you are hardheaded, strong-willed, and stubborn like I once was, it will be more difficult. You will get knocked down more times than you could ever imagine until you reach that moment when all seems lost, when you finally give up, let go, and surrender because it is too painful to go on. In these moments, you may feel defeated, but you are not. You are finally ready to put an end to the cycle and evolve so that it never recurs in your life again. This is the point in your life where experiencing pain, in its finality, will transform you in more beautiful ways.

Whatever form trauma arrives in, feeling your way through it is the only way through it. The evolution of your soul hinges on it. When traumatic events happen, our world crumbles, and time stands still. We become frozen by the circumstances that have violated us in a painful way, rather than seeing the meaning behind the event—yet there is always a greater meaning behind each of these events. Seeing them for what they truly are, grasping the lessons they are trying to teach you, and understanding the grounds from which they have grown will help you overcome them with stronger will and determination as you continue to evolve and grow.

Recurring Themes

For me, these lessons appeared three times over 20 years. The events lasted longer and were more painful each time. I could see the commonality in all three experiences, and by the third, I could finally see what they were all trying to teach me. Valuable lessons that were imperative to my growth and my future. My happiness was solely dependent on me learning these lessons. When I finally did, I experienced true happiness in a form I had never felt before. The beauty in this was that once I learned these lessons, I finally knew that I would never repeat them, nor would I even entertain the idea of them any longer. I knew that I would no longer manifest this type of experience in my life or the kind of people involved in them. That in itself gave me an enormous sense of peace. It is one of the many beautiful gifts that learning these lessons will give you. It will also give you the self-confidence needed to move forward in your life, self-confidence that you may have believed was missing from your life before now.

At that point, that inner knowingness that had been pulling at me for decades finally liberated me to trust the Universe and follow its guidance. When I finally understood the true meaning behind the lessons that I needed to learn and not the definition I was giving them, I reevaluated my life going back to a time before these events presented themselves to me. I wanted to go back to the beginning of my life to try to understand where the imbalances occurred that were tormenting me well into my 20s, 30s, and 40s. I had to know, understand, and heal these areas of my being. This was the only way to release these heavy emotions and ensure they would not return. I was diligent and engaged in pursuing this knowledge, and I was committed to finding answers. I was gracious, kind, and patient with myself during this time and gave myself the grace I desperately needed to see this through. Grace was something I had always given to others but not to myself—one of the many lessons I needed to learn.

Healing through Trauma

When the healing from my trauma began, I kept reflecting on the works of Brian L. Weiss, M.D. I had read all his books over the last 30 years and had always been drawn to his work, which involved past-life regressions and healing. I knew that I was an old soul, and I also knew that some of these connections I carried into this life were from lives before this one, many of which I wanted to understand so that I could put closure on them and release them. I needed to close these chapters of my life because they were holding me back from the life I had desired and wanted. I knew Dr. Weiss was no longer working one-on-one with clients, so I began focusing on healing the wounds I had felt so deeply and releasing them from my body myself. Then another miracle was presented to me—in the divine timing of the Universe, of course. You will see as you begin this journey how magic begins to unfold all around you *(smiling)*. You will be supported in many beautiful and profound ways.

I received a call from my cousin Lorenzo and his wife, Kellie, who were preparing to move back to London. During our call, Kellie began telling me about a friend from Ireland—a woman named Triona Sheeran. Triona is a clinical and spiritual hypnotherapist specializing in QHHT° (Level 3)—Quantum Healing Hypnosis Technique—and Lives Between Lives regression therapy. I was excited but not surprised, as that was how my life had unfolded since November 2022. I knew that I needed to speak with Triona. I knew she would help me uncover the mystery behind some of the emotions I was feeling that I could not trace back to a source in this life. I knew that I needed to go much deeper than conventional therapy, and I knew that a past-life regression was what I needed to complete my journey into healing. It had fascinated me all my life, for good reason, and now it was magically appearing in my life when I needed it most. You will begin to see this happening in your life as you move through your transformation *(smiling)*.

Once again, I took a leap of faith and contacted Triona. Triona and I began conversing about her work and my journey. I was fascinated by her and knew that this was someone whom I needed to work with. We scheduled my first session with her remotely. Strangely enough, I was not nervous about this. I was excited. If something deeply rooted within me was holding me back, I wanted to uncover it and release it. Heal from it. I knew that knowing the truth, in whichever form it came to me, was the only way through. I wanted to know where this would take me in my healing journey, as it was entering my life in perfect timing for a reason. I also wanted closure to a connection that had been a source of great pain for me over the last two decades: a person I had believed was so much more than they indeed were. One of the greatest disappointments of my life and the most heartbreaking was because this person was not living his truth; instead, he lived within the facade that he had built to hide behind. His truth would have been a far greater choice had he had the courage to follow through. It would have brought him a life of love and happiness had he had the courage to go within and do this work. I had met many people like this throughout my life, and this was something I no longer wanted in my life. I wanted to be free of all people like this, as all the betrayal, heartbreak, and pain I had experienced had come from people like this—people who were unwilling to see the truth and pave a new way for themselves. People I trusted, gave my heart and soul to, made every sacrifice imaginable for, who were utterly deceptive. I wanted to try to understand what it was within me that was so completely shattered as to allow this to happen. This was now at the forefront of my life—healing my grief, my trauma, and the part of me that manifested such losses in my life.

If you are a giver, like I was, give to yourself first and foremost. Once you do, you will see that the individuals who took so much from you will be released from your life. You never needed them, even when you believed that you did. You can still give of yourself, only now it will be to people who come into your life with the same beautiful intentions as you and who will reciprocate your efforts—one of the beautiful lessons of learning to give *and receive.*

Past-Life Regressions

The morning of my first session with Triona was now upon me. I was surprisingly calm and not at all skeptical. The Universe guided her to me, and I trusted that. I knew this experience would deepen my understanding of many things. In all the books I have read about past-life regressions, I was always amazed by how quickly healing occurred by understanding the source of pain at such a deep level. I was unsure how this would work for me or *if* it would work for me, but I was open to it and hopeful.

As soon as I connected with Triona, I loved her. She has a very calming and angelic presence about her that I could feel and sense immediately. I instantly relaxed and let my guard down. I felt completely safe and at peace going through this journey with her. We spoke in depth for the first part of our call, and then she asked me if I wanted to begin my first past-life regression. I did, and we started.

During this session, I was lying in bed and very relaxed. Triona began by taking me into an even more relaxed state of consciousness. I was aware of everything that was happening and open to it.

I was conscious about being conscious, if that makes sense *(smiling)*. She gently guided me in a way that allowed me to go deep within. With her help, I journeyed into five past lives. It was incredible. With each life, I could physically feel the person I was, the rooms I was in, the places I lived, and the emotions I felt in those moments. Some experiences brought me to tears, and others brought me great joy. As I was experiencing each past life, I could feel my heart healing in a way I did not believe possible until now. Before this, my heart was heavy and blocked, unemotional and afraid to feel. This work opened me up in a way that I needed. In each life, I was of different ages and in different bodies, but there were some similarities between those lives and this one. That was where the messages were for me, and I was absorbing it all. They were so vivid and so real, unexplainable, and miraculous. In one vision, I was an infant born to an emotionally unavailable and narcissistic mother. I was more of a prize possession to her that gave her credibility and stature than a child she brought into this life to love, cherish, and protect. I could see that this was where so many of my issues of self-worth, self-love, safety, and vulnerability came from. It also made me understand why I am so overly loving to my own children, as I never want them to feel unloved, unprotected, and uncherished by me—I want to give them a healthy, loving, and stable foundation above all else. I have always wanted this for them, as I never felt like I had it, even though I was born into a very loving and stable family. It was clear that these feelings I had been living with and struggling with did not come from this lifetime. I brought them with me to heal and evolve away from, as I was manifesting them in many ways in this life.

At the end of this session with Triona, I saw a glimpse of something that gave me such hope and so much healing all at the same time. I woke from this journey with a much deeper understanding of myself and the parts of me that needed healing the most—my trauma. I felt my body healing from these repeating experiences in my life. The teachers in these lessons served a great purpose. I could see them clearly and differently now. Not as friends, family, or even loved ones but for who and what they were to me in my journey into

Emotional Wellness

healing. I could clearly see how damaged people damaged others. And this is what they did to me, but not to destroy me, even though many things did. It was to evolve me. Lessons I needed to learn to live a much happier and fulfilling life. It was part of their journey, too, and one day it will be part of their healing, should they choose to evolve. It is a choice we all have to make in our life. You cannot make this choice for them; you can only make it for yourself and hold space in your heart for them to do the same. As devastating as it may feel to release these people from your life, you must. It is the only way through.

Healing from Trauma Is a Process

Whole-body healing includes healing from loss, grief, and trauma. In life, these events are inevitable. We will all experience all these intense emotions throughout our lives. Though they will all be different for everyone, healing through these emotions is vital to the life we wish to live. It is a process and not one that you can rush through, avoid, or deny, for if you do, you will carry its remnants with you throughout your lifetime until you heal. In some cases, you can bring it into this life from past lives, which was one lesson I learned in my past-life regressions when certain emotions did not feel like anything I experienced in this life. Understanding this is life-changing.

Some massive events happened to me throughout my life and my healing journey. Some were so incredibly painful that they set me back weeks, months, and years. I allowed these heavy feelings and emotions to control my every move. I was lost within them and honestly did not know where to begin, as it was all so overwhelming, especially during the worst of my illness. I did what I did best: I buried myself in my work and buried these strong emotions and feelings as deeply as possible until I was ready to process them. It wasn't until my father passed away that I truly understood what it meant to heal, as I was so shattered, broken, and on the precipice of my life. I could not see a way out of my pain other than succumbing to it and finally feeling my way through it. I knew I needed to

91

release decades of all I was carrying with me. I spent the next 10 months focused on this work and dealing with every emotion I had ever buried within me.

I saw these events as the turning points in my life, leading me back to my truth, my soul's purpose.

Trauma is different for everyone, and patience, grace, and kindness are essential. Whether you are grieving or someone you love is grieving from trauma, it is part of your journey and unavoidable. My father passed away after nine months of hospice and crisis care during the most crucial moments of my life. I was unprepared for the pain that I would feel. It felt unbearable at times. I dedicated myself to understanding why this was all happening at once. What did I most need to learn about myself, life, death, and how holistic health and wellness throughout life played a vital and irreplaceable role in all of it? My commitment to understanding and healing led me through.

Uncovering the Beauty in the Trauma

It may be difficult to imagine that there can be beauty in the depths of trauma, heartbreak, grief, devastation, and loss, but as with all things that break us, they also revive us, redefine us, and recreate us; that is where beauty emerges. When you can look back at everything you have been through with a kind and gentle heart, you will understand that you have evolved into the beautiful light within you. These solid and painful emotions are not there to derail us from our soul's purpose, even though they do momentarily. They teach us and guide us back to who we are and not the facade created by escaping them. Face them with a valiant heart and uncover your life's beauty and magic. It is there, and it is waiting for you.

Nothing outside of ourselves will make us whole or complete. You are already complete. Listen to the messages and heal your mind, heart, soul, and body. Your life will be so much better for it, and you already know that *(smiling)*.

• • •

My Past-Life Regression

These are some revelations I experienced from my first regression session with Triona and her professional analysis of our session together. Through my success, my dedication, my diligence, and raising my beautiful children, it was easy at first to ignore the telltale signs of the trauma I had been carrying throughout my life. Each time I was triggered, they surfaced again and again, only much more robust and profound within me until I did this work. My triggers no longer trigger me.

After the heartbreak and the loss of my father, heartbreak and loss mixed with complex grief felt unbearable; I made the choice not to bury it but to face it head-on. I was unsure where to begin regarding past-life regressions and reincarnation, especially the therapeutic side of regression therapy. I felt a pull to it, an internal recognition that this trauma (grief) and so much more were directing many areas of my life and life choices. I sometimes thought I had no control over it, but I found out I did by healing it. I followed my intuition without question, and the result was, once again, beautiful.

I knew deep within my soul that this was the trauma that I had carried over from another life, surfacing repeatedly. I wanted to, and needed to, eradicate it from my body so it could be healed and released. I had to end it, so I took action as I was intuitively guided to.

During my regression therapy session with Triona, I didn't have to think about where to go as the scenes unfolded all around me and all on their own, first as a young woman and then into another life as an older woman. After that life, I could look back and see how it all connected to my life in this lifetime. The lessons I did not learn then carried over into this life to be learned.

It also showed me how often I did not have boundaries as an empath. I spent most of my life putting other people and their needs before mine. It was clear that self-love was one of the many lessons in this life that I needed to learn and embrace. I realized how many relationships I was involved in where this theme and pattern were prevalent. I could see it so clearly upon waking up from this session.

Discovering the truth behind your trauma, acknowledging it, and facing it are the most essential ways to release these deep and heavy emotions from your body and heal from them. These are feelings and emotions that you do not want to carry with you throughout your lifetime or into your next. Becoming aware of all my subconscious limitations, trauma, or triggers was so healing for me, and it gave me a sense of self-empowerment to be fully present with who I AM, not as others see me or who I am to them, but for ME as ME. These emotions no longer defined me or my life.

When I connected to this light within me even deeper, it felt like home. It felt like I was one with my body and at peace. Over the next week, I continued to process information and expand my journey. We are all together in this big, beautiful, magical puzzle that we call life. No one can escape it, especially when you have a much larger calling in life as you have, and it is time to embrace that truth. You would not have gone through all that you have if you did not. I know you know this too. You must now clear away the triggers and emotions holding you back. Living consciously is how all these pieces come together and make perfect sense, as you will see by doing this work.

Trauma, grief, pain, sorrow, shame, remorse, and guilt are all to be experienced in this life. I reflected upon this, not only on my journey but also my friends and relationships. We are all here to experience an array of emotions, feel them, share them, see them, and then choose to let them go. It is a choice. And it is worth making, as it will completely release you from the hold they once had over you and your life.

It will give you strength, and it will make you whole.

Notes on Valentina's Session

BY TRIONA SHEERAN

Trauma is a word that most people have heard of, but not every-one always understands.

Trauma is the part of the brain that understands emotions, holding on to specific events and memories, as it feels it is protect-ing the person from experiencing pain again. It makes perfect sense, except, when experiencing this pain, it is precisely what the soul needs to continue to evolve. Dolores Cannon, a pioneer in her field, says that "Earth is a learning school," meaning we choose to experi-ence trauma to understand all emotions better.

We often see things from a more internal viewpoint (under-standable, as it can be challenging to experience emotional pain sometimes). Still, if we step back, it can become much more appar-ent that this trauma we experienced in our past is more of a learning experience, just like a child who falls with a shoe untied will learn to tie their shoes the next time.

Metaphysically speaking, much trauma is carried in the body, as the long-term memory (subconscious) holds and stores mem-ory but does not understand time. Something experienced in child-hood, the womb, or another lifetime is still very prevalent in this lifetime, and we can usually feel it in the body. It is one aspect of metaphysical anatomy.

We can carry trauma from another life to this lifetime to help work through life themes or lessons. The major life themes that the majority of people work on are:

Self-love, self-esteem, self-confidence, boundaries, shame, guilt, and grief.

Which ones are your lessons to learn in this lifetime?

It can take one lifetime or many to understand it and then let it go entirely.

We choose to experience these lessons for the most part, and then we are supposed to decide to let them go, but as you know, life can be a little more complex, and thus, free will leads us to carry them a little longer (or much longer) than we need to. We are manifesting in our actions, our thoughts, our energy, our health, and our well-being.

As Valentina explains what happened to her, we can deeply feel past-life trauma and childhood trauma that even our cells hold on to, that hers held on to.

Trauma can be the simplest of memories (falling off a bike) or more complex grief, abandonment, and abuse (physical and emotional). The deeper we feel it, the more it is repeated, and the stronger it becomes.

As divine beings of light, we are all connected through our higher selves; in all essence, we feel each other's pain to some degree. We collectively experience many life lessons together. In our life plans or soul contracts, we share life events and relationships that will encourage us to face these traumas and life lessons so we can remove them (think soul growth and its primary purpose to continue to learn).

A trigger is when you consciously are not aware of trauma but you have a response anyway to a person or an event, smell, or even a sound.

The part of you that always remembers things in the now (the long-term memory) reflects and is triggered by one of the above. So we agree that various people and situations come into our lives at different times to help us see, feel, and remove them.

A lot of our brain power and energy goes into feeding the trauma, so it is hugely rewarding in our minds and bodies to let it go.

I met Valentina through a mutual friend; her energy immediately felt right. You know the slight chill that runs up your spine and the goose bumps you get when something resonates with you? I trust those physical signs, knowing my higher self or guides tell me to pay attention.

I was not surprised that Valentina was a very enlightened soul, full of compassion and heartfelt generosity. The light was beaming from her. She was knowledgeable about all aspects of mind, body, and spirit, which means, me being me, I could talk to her all day long.

In the first discussion, which is a preinterview for a session, we discussed how she was feeling.

Frustrated—Disheartened—Taken for granted

Situations were arising around her that triggered how she gives so much of herself and sometimes for very little or nothing in return. Being the compassionate, kind soul she is, it would not even bother her except it bothered her subconscious mind as one of Valentina's main life lessons in this lifetime. Self-love. With self-love as a life theme, people (relationships, family, colleagues) will continuously and unconsciously trigger that within you to help you remove it.

It is prevalent for so many healers and empaths like Valentina. They want to do whatever they can to help to the detriment of their own energy.

After the first interview, I knew she needed to love herself first and foremost at the most apparent bubble or trigger of being taken for granted and self-love. We decided on a past-life regression. I do various other modalities like empowerment sessions, trauma release, and QHHT, which are always in person. The distance being an issue at the time, we decided on a past-life regression using RT (regression therapy). We later did a QHHT session in New York City, which was amazing as I met her in person. So beautiful and inspiring. A light in her own right.

Back to her first session. It is always the intention for one past life only, which is very important, as we genuinely want to clear this trauma or unwanted program and energy block, and the best way to do this is to embody it, which is one lifetime.

From the start, Valentina was most unusual: a 15-minute induction turned into four minutes, as she was already in a lifetime before I could even count her down—I could see from her energy and altered states as she started to talk about "an older body in an unfamiliar place."

Going with the client's energy is always an excellent therapeutic decision, so we explored various scenes and essential days. Valentina was the exception, not the rule, as she instead decided to jump into different lifetimes instead of other events in the one life; for the most part, we explored them in detail and then, putting on my therapist hat, I brought her back to the most important one.

The healing was seeing how important it was to let go—to love oneself unconditionally no matter what—to stay in her power.

We did some transformational healing by using the part of the mind that is open for direct suggestions (subconscious), and we inputted some wanted programs to help move her forward.

Valentina visited the source light and her higher self, where she was reminded how powerful she is and how powerful we all are as individuals and collective beings. It gave her hope to continue on her journey, have clarity, and know that she is never alone and is always supported.

Events That Bring On Trauma and Their Triggers

In their essence, traumatic events can come in many ways, most of which begin in childhood. They could be from an absent parent, an alcoholic parent, physical, emotional, and verbal abuse, sexual abuse, bullying, family additions, abandonment, hospital- or health-related, pressure to overperform and achieve and not to fail. They can surface in many ways in your life: via addiction (work included), fears, phobias, low self-esteem, depression, chronic anxiety, inability to express feelings and emotions (emotionally unavailable), and anger. Triggers can manifest in resentment, anger, rumination, and feeling shaken within your body. These are just some of the ways that trauma can present itself in your life, but no matter what form it arrives in, you can feel your way through it, heal from it, and release it from your body. This will transform your life in profound ways as you will see as you begin to heal from any trauma that you might be carrying with you as it is time to let it go.

Your Trauma

Have you experienced trauma, grief, loss, heartbreak, betrayal, or any abuse (physical or emotional)? Can you identify if these events are recurring events in your life? Can you identify the life lessons that these events are teaching you?

Were these smaller events that spanned over the course of your life or massive events that have occurred all at once? How did you respond to them? Did you face them and feel your way through the pain of them, or did you suppress them?

Have these events resulted in lasting triggers that have sabotaged situations in your life in ways that may not be in your best interest? Have you identified these triggers?

Once you define these events and triggers, can you feel your way through them (if you have not already), heal from them, and release them with love and understanding?

Can you find peace within yourself as you move through these emotions? Can you see their beauty through the life lessons they have taught and are teaching you?

Can you define what your life lessons are in this lifetime?

Once you define them, can you begin to heal these parts of yourself so that you can embrace the life meant for you? The **love** *meant for you?*

Chapter Ten

LOVE

The Valiant Heart and the Relationships We Embody

Love . . . it surrounds every being
and extends slowly to embrace all that shall be.

— KHALIL GIBRAN

Love. It is the most beautiful experience that this life has to offer us. It comes in many forms and ways, and we are the source of it in our lives. What you believe about love, you manifest. So let us clear the pathways to the love that you desire.

The Most Important Relationship, the One with Ourselves

Love is beautiful, soulful, and inspiring. It is graceful, kind, gentle, and patient, and it is precisely what your soul needs in more ways than one. Love is something that we tend to give to others so passionately, so willingly, so easily, and so intentionally. Yet when it comes to loving ourselves and our bodies, our soul's true protector and guide, we do not love or cherish them so quickly and so effortlessly, especially during life's challenges. Instead of seeing all the beauty and magic that we are made of and encompass, we tend to look at ourselves with blame, shame, and sometimes even contempt and self-loathing. I know that I did, and you most likely have too.

When I was at my worst, there were times when I could not even look at myself in the mirror, let alone accept what I was seeing. I was unrecognizable to myself in every way. The reflection that looked back upon me was a stranger I did not know or wish to know. At times I disassociated from myself because I could no longer bear the painful sight of the mental, emotional, and physical changes that were happening to me, changes I believed at the time I had no control over and could not understand for the life of me. No one could. In those moments, which were more like years, I felt hopeless and alone.

I had loved many parts of myself throughout my life, yet I could not muster up the same kind of love and respect for myself when I needed it the most. I did not know or understand how that could ever change. I was drowning in the emotions of all that my illness was taking away from me that I had cherished my entire life and, in many ways, taken for granted. I took for granted that I would always have endless energy, a vital existence, a strong body, long, thick, beautiful hair, my love for life, and so much more. The list was endless. I could no longer be the beautiful, desirable, passionate, or lovable person my husband had fallen in love with or the adoring mother to my children that I had always been. So I isolated myself from everyone but my immediate family.

I did not wish to be around people, or to be touched, or even to be looked at. I wanted to be left alone to deal with all the emotions consuming me. I could not find the space or the words for my loved ones. I was suffocating, and I was suffering. I worked from home as much as possible and went into my studios when classes were not in session so I would not have to see anyone physically. I became antisocial in search of answers. Until I began this work, I had not stopped to consider that my thoughts about my body contributed to my ailments. I stopped supporting it in the way that I once had. I stopped working out, which used to be my daily ritual. I was emotionally eating and not fueling my body with the nutrient-rich and soul-loving foods that I was accustomed to. I took out all my frustrations and emotions on my body as if it were the culprit. At this moment in my life, loving myself was not an option for me, though it should have been, as it is a vital element of healing.

I did not want to embody, feel, or give love—a condition that was far from who I was naturally. Love was all that I had ever lived for. It was my energy force my entire life. It inspired me, drove me, and was what I had genuinely embodied before my illness. When I lost that magic from my life that used to radiate from within me so brightly, I should have realized that something was seriously wrong. I felt like my body had betrayed me somehow, and I was living in the mindset that I would never again feel the love for myself or for anyone else, other than my children, that I once did. It was deeply disheartening for me. At the same time, this feeling also became a monumental part of my healing journey. Even though I had buried the magic that I had once had, there was always this flame dimly lit deep within me that I knew was still there. I was denying it, but it was always there.

During times of crisis, we tend to betray ourselves the most with our inner critiques rather than supporting ourselves through the crisis lovingly and kindly. As I dove deeper into this inner work, I could see how showing myself and my body a much deeper love than ever before was very healing. I began to see that my body was not failing me, attacking me, or betraying me. It was simply sending me the most profound and life-changing messages in the only way it could. My body showed me, through illness, that I was not aligned with my heart, my soul, and my soul's purpose. My soul chose this body for a purpose, and it was not aligned with that purpose, so it guided me back to my inner self, where my light was still shining. I would have preferred a much simpler method of awakening, but then I realized I'd missed all of them the first time around *(smiling)*. You will not have to.

I had been focusing outward when I needed to be focusing inward. The inner critique that tormented me was of my own making; now it would have to be reckoned with and conquered, and love was the only way through this. Love got me through it—love of self. I could not see that at the time, but I can now. Clearly.

Each step brought me closer and closer to a much deeper love for my soul than I had ever known. As my mindset started to shift, my thoughts became more loving and encouraging, which filled my heart with hope. As I accepted all of the choices I had made and the people I allowed into my life who caused me such strife,

I could finally let go, forgive, and move on from all of them with love, ensuring that they would not return again in any way. I was done with them. With each step I courageously took to overcome my fears and finally face them, I became even stronger in my body. Releasing decades and even centuries of trauma *(smiling)* set my soul free from so much pain that I was carrying and had been storing within my body. Just waking up to my truth was all it took for me to understand and comprehend the source of my pain, especially in my body. I could then release it from my body, ensuring that it would not take its hold over me once again. It was all so essential to my healing. Love. I knew that significant shifts in my life were forthcoming, and when I was ready, divine guidance stepped in and brought it all to light for me, and it will for you too.

I was forever changed when I reached this point of self-love. I knew that I would not return to that place where I had come from ever again. I was committed. I had to be. It felt too incredible to turn back. Healing was happening, and self-love was in everything I did. I loved myself, but now it was time to face my body. With my armor on, I was now ready to surrender. The white flag was up. I love anything and everything white, so this was a fabulous white dress for me. Once again I was thinking superficially and not realizing that all the work I was committed to was transforming my body through it all. You will be amazed at how beautifully your body will begin to transform once you learn to love it and genuinely love it.

As I was releasing so much that my body had been carrying, the weight I had held on to as protection throughout this time was releasing itself from me too. My body was transforming, as was my life. My body and soul were aligning again, and I was becoming whole. I was beginning to truly understand that my body was guiding me back to love all this time. It was not gentle, but it was necessary. I was finally listening to my body once again. It had been guiding me through this journey so I could heal my inner self. Intimately and patiently, I was opening my heart from its deep sleep and feeling so much love and revival. It was, and still is, all-consuming. I was returning to love. Love in my heart and all things was an essential part of this. I realized that by only loving myself at my best and not when it needed me the most, I was causing more pain within myself. I am no longer that stubborn and prideful person that I once was. The lightheartedness that I feel now is something I cherish. I will protect it with all my might, and you will too.

Creating Healthy Boundaries

Creating healthy boundaries is a sign of love for yourself first and foremost. You will begin to protect your peace of mind and well-being at all costs once you see how much of yourself you have lost to other people's needs and requirements. It will become very clear to you who needs to be released from your life, and you will release them. My father always told me to leave people better than I found them, and I have lived by that, but now it was time to do this for me, and I did. It was not and is not a selfish act but a necessary one. It is best to release them so they can grow and evolve as they are meant to. They taught you what they came into your life to teach you, and you will have done the same in return. Love yourself and them enough to let them go. This journey will teach you that you cannot heal another person's soul; they must do this work for themselves when they are ready. This time is all about you and your healing.

I released so many people who were only taking from me. People who did not appreciate all I had given them from a place of love and nothing more. It was always the way for me. It brought me so much joy to give and give and give and make everyone's life that much easier. I do not regret that part of my personality. I am still very much a giving and generous person, but it is for the people I choose to allow into my life whom I feel deserve to be in it and reciprocate my kindness, as it is the only way forward for me now. People who disrespect you, disappear from your life, or cannot be truly honest with you are people whom you do not want in your life. They hide behind a facade and are cowards at best. They are the people who benefited from you and acted as if you had no part in it. You know, those who take credit for your brilliance and hard work and treat you as an option versus who you truly are—a superpower *(smiling)!* You will find great solace in releasing them from your life. It is also a grand gesture of love of self.

Relationships of the Heart

As beautiful as you are and are becoming through this journey, you will begin to surround yourself with individuals who are as evolved as you and continue to grow with you. You will love yourself enough to shield yourself from anything else. Superficial relationships will not excite you, and you will not wish to engage in them any longer.

One of the most beautiful and desirable elements of loving yourself is the intimacy that comes with it. One can only share their depth deeply with another through truth, grace, and completeness. Loving yourself is all of those things and so much more. A beautiful relationship can flourish when two people share in their entirety and do not need to complete one another. Healing is a journey, but loving yourself is a gift you give yourself and those you love. Everyone must do this work for themselves from a place of love, *and our soul embodies this kind of love.*

Sharing this kind of love with someone is a gift that can only be reciprocated by someone who understands this and who has begun their own inner work to meet you where you are. In this way, you will continue to evolve and grow together, the only way for two souls to prosper passionately within the depths of love. This is a love that words alone cannot truly express, as it is to be experienced and felt within your heart and soul. Anything less than this and you will always find yourself longing, which is why this work is so special, because it takes you to that place within you where you are already enough and loved so deeply that the person who meets you at this place will share in it with you. It will be a beautiful and undeniable synergy of energies—love beyond anything you could imagine.

You will know this love because it will meet you fearlessly, truthfully, lovingly, and passionately, and you will be ready for it and prepared to meet it. It will be without fears, distractions, manipulations, mind games, and all those other things that people who are not yet healed tend to do. You will be a priority as they will be to you. It will be a natural flow of energy between you because you will both feel safe within who you are and within one another.

This kind of love comes from a place of peace shared with another—deeply intimate conversations versus messaging via text. I say this because so many people engage in relationships via text, which is unsustainable. You cannot build a beautiful, loving, intimate, and soulful foundation based on messaging in this way, nor should you. This form of communication is inadequate at best. It is devoid of all intimacy in every way. Intimacy and intimate moments are experienced and expressed in so many beautiful ways when present and heard. They are not something you will fear or need to hide behind.

Your heart and soul will manifest the most beautiful relationship for you when doing this work, built on being present, loving, graceful, supportive, intimate, passionate, generous, and kind. Abundant in all ways. You will not experience it any other way, nor would you desire to. This does exist for you; it is coming if it has not already.

If I had it to do all over again, I would do it from a place of love through all of it. It would have changed everything. It would have made my experience less painful and my recovery much quicker. I am convinced of this now. Love, in all its beauty, is the only way through life as we know it and will come to know it.

Love yourself, as you are beautiful!

Your Love

As you look back upon your life and those you have loved,
friends, and family, can you see where, had you loved yourself first
and foremost, you would have made different choices?

Can you see where you felt taken for granted or misled
in some way that benefited the person but not you, leaving you hurt
or feeling abandoned? Can you see where having healthy boundaries
could have served you well and will serve you well now?

When you look at your life and the relationships it embodies,
are they loving, intimate, and passionate, and do they make you feel safe,
protected, supported, and at peace? If they do not, are you ready
to release them, trusting that the right relationships will
enter your life now because they will?

There is so much love that awaits you. Love yourself beyond **belief.**

part iv

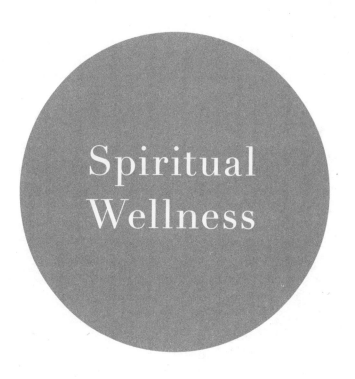

Spiritual
Wellness

Chapter Eleven

BELIEF

Beyond the Physical Body

*The appearance of things changes according to the emotions;
and thus we see magic and beauty in them, while the
magic and beauty are really in ourselves.*

— KAHLIL GIBRAN

Belief in the unknown embodies courage, gallantry, and humbleness within the absence of fear, pridefulness, and ego. It is significant, as it embraces the mindset that we are limitless and boundless within this Universe. It transcends our self-inflicted limitations, insecurities, and preconceived notions about ourselves. It is an exquisite and delicate balance between being consciously receptive and being grounded in reason, allowing for exploration and self-discovery without succumbing to the unreasonable idea that we are limited by what is known to us or scientifically proven to be so.

Belief beyond Our Physical Realities

This chapter is about belief, not in a religious sense, but in a soul sense. The confidence that surfaces within our physical bodies goes beyond what our minds can truly comprehend or understand; it escapes all reason and logic. It is the inner knowingness that works this way: in the moments you feel it, you *know*. You do not understand how you know, but you know precisely without questions or explanation. We have these moments all the time, and until we are ready, we dismiss them only to find out later (sometimes much later) that the feeling we had felt initially, and so profoundly, was precise.

Sometimes it is a sense exhilarating you with feelings of happiness, peace, beauty, and joy that light you up from the inside out and beautifully invigorate your entire body and soul. Sometimes it is a feeling that makes you feel uncomfortable, fearful, anxious, and unsafe in your surroundings, a not-so-delicate warning from the Universe. It is your soul guiding you through your physical senses. **Your intuition.** It is more potent than anything else in your life. It is your life force. Your energy force. Your guiding light. If you believe in it, your life will evolve magically, taking you beyond your most profound dreams, expectations, and imaginations for yourself and your soul's purpose.

This sense. This voice. This inner knowingness will take you where you wish to go if you can find it within yourself to listen, trust, and have faith in it genuinely. It will not harm you; it will only protect you. As your body begins to heal and you begin to do this inner work, you will notice this more and more. You may have begun to notice it already, so you may already know what I am speaking of. Our bodies are miraculous in this way and in their ability to heal and guide us, but we must open ourselves up to this gift and remain open to what it is trying to tell us, and then we must trust in it enough to allow it to guide us. You can trust your body. You can trust your soul. You can trust its guidance wholeheartedly and with every ounce of your being. It is there for you and you only, as it is you in your most immaculate form.

Our intuitive nature is powerful, and it is integral to our lives. This inner knowingness silently speaks and draws us toward our greatest gifts. It guides us throughout our journey—if only we would trust in it enough to listen to it the first time we hear it—in a way that is so much deeper than we can comprehend or even describe with words, written or spoken. It is home to our authentic brilliance and intelligence. Our mastery over everything we seek to enjoy. It is our soul speaking to us and through us. Our mission, purpose, and ability to see and feel beyond the physical elements of our life. It is our inner wisdom; if we believe in it with all our heart and soul, we will avoid all that tries to derail us from our most abundant self and lives, including heartache and heartbreak. It is that precise. It is one of the greatest lessons of this lifetime. It is what unites us in one commonality that connects us all. We all have our lessons to learn, but this one, we all share in—the oneness within our mind, heart, soul, and body, living consciously within their knowledge, wisdom, and guidance.

It is your birthright.

We are all born with this incredible and undeniable gift. This inner knowingness that we are born with is our birthright to guide us throughout our lifetime. It is precise and will not misguide you if you trust in it wholeheartedly and fearlessly, without ego or fear or the will to deny it, avoid it, and sabotage it, as that brings unhappiness, despair, anxiety, depression, illness, and a life unfulfilled. It truly is your choice. No one else can make it for you. If you allow others to, you will lose your way and lose yourself in someone else's journey. This journey of healing is yours and yours alone. Beyond your physical body and mind is your pathway toward belief. Believe in the magic of your inner knowingness. It is wondrous at heart and holds the key to your true happiness.

Your soul is everlasting, eternal, and endless. Your soul existed before this body, and your soul will continue to exist after this body, as your soul is ageless and timeless. Though your body will age and change, your soul will move through your many lives unchanging and enduring. We cannot deny these changes even though we do our best to try and deny their existence by silencing them until we are ready to accept them. If you think about the years leading up to this one, you will understand this. You have aged, your body has aged, you have become wiser and more aware, and you have evolved, yet your soul has been the eternal force within you, unaltered by your external circumstances. It will always feel supportive in energy as it guides you toward your reawakening. It is time to trust it, believe in it, have faith in its guidance, and fearlessly and openly follow its lead. Your soul will protect you if you allow it to. In the good times and the not-so-good, it will always guide you and lead you back to your heart's and soul's deepest desires, your purpose in this life.

Your soul is eternal. Your soul will empower you with its infinite and ancient wisdom that you have access to consciously and unconsciously whenever you need it, but would it not be most genuinely fabulous to live within it consciously versus living without it or denying it? Yes, it would. It holds all the answers to all of your questions. It truly does, like nothing outside yourself ever could. This is your birthright, as you were born with it.

The Power of Belief

Belief is powerful. It will bring you love, understanding, compassion, and completeness. You will no longer feel a longing for anything outside of yourself, as you will know and feel complete within. Everything that is for you will be divinely guided toward you in its own perfect time. Your heart will be free from all fear and will only feel love for all that you encounter. You will have a greater understanding that you are not alone and that you are protected and safe. Love will return to you more profoundly, as you will see it and feel it in everything, even all that you believed you could not overcome as you have, and you will. Belief is a powerful thing, and it is yours to believe in. I can say all of this because this is how it happened to me. Beyond what I could then comprehend, it happened and it has remained a constant force within my life.

At the center of belief, you will find serenity, the tranquil recognition that despite our many efforts, advancements, programming, and accumulated knowledge, there is yet so much that is still unknown to us, going way beyond the grasp of human understanding and acknowledgment. By acknowledging that our current state of understanding our reality is merely a glance at the vast tapestry of our existence, you can approach the unknown with wonder and grace, opening yourself to these new revelations, infinite possibilities, and innovational and imaginative breakthroughs that challenge the existing paradigms of your life.

Courage and wonder make great companions in this journey toward a much deeper and more meaningful life. They help you face uncertainty with an unwavering soul, fearless in its belief in the unknown. Belief is your ability and willingness to shift out of the darkness that surrounds you, guided by your curiosity in search of more knowledge. Knowledge that you know exists for you beyond what you already understand and have accepted as your truth. It does not diminish or deny the presence of fear in these moments; it simply acknowledges it, yet the choice is to move forward despite it. It is your commitment to evolution, healing, and enlightenment, even when the path seems mysterious, unclear, and uncertain.

Belief is without ego.

The ego has no real place in your life. It prevents you from moving forward, as you must, by creating barriers and obstacles that hold you back from becoming truly authentic, present, and fully engaged in your life and in the great unknown. It solely survives on the need to be correct and inserts itself as the ultimate truth when, in reality, it is far from the truth. It is limiting, and it is a limiting belief. Ultimately, it leads you to believe that the truth cannot truly be known to you because it cannot penetrate the barricades that your ego has built around the truth. Eliminating the ego mindset from your life liberates you from the limitations and personal prejudices that it set for your life, which allows you to flourish within your quest for greater knowledge and understanding. Eliminating it will open you up to embrace the endless possibilities for yourself and your life, for profound transformation. It will lift the veil so you can clearly see and understand the enigmas, paradoxes, and ambiguities that have held you captive all this time via your ego.

Belief is the culmination of science, spirituality, logic, and intuition. A place where they all rendezvous and converge in ways that defy reason and interpretation. By embracing the mystery and intimacy of these elements, we create a sacred space for a more holistic gateway to understanding the world in which we exist.

Believing in the Wonderment of the Unknown

Believing in the unknown without fear and ego is being present, living in the moments of your life. It involves humility, courage, and an open heart. It is the recognition of the limitations that you have placed on yourself while nurturing a passionate desire to rise above those limitations and boundaries. It invites you to explore the depths of your existence with wonder, curiosity, and resilience as you engage in all you discover within yourself. It is like dancing on the precipice of the mysterious while finding beauty and wisdom in the monumental and majestic magnitude of the unknown that beautifully vibrates throughout our bodies in wonderment and awe.

Belief and wonderment are then beautifully intertwined and woven throughout our experiences. Guiding us throughout our journey of exploration and understanding ourselves and the Universe in which we live. Together, they are essential in our intellectual and emotional engagements, inviting us to accept the known with the unknown with absolute certainty. As you have come to know, understand, and accept everything known to you, trust in the unknown in the same way. Belief is not motionless; it evolves as we evolve. It is the willingness to remain open even when challenges arise from opposing forces and views within us or by others. Alternatively, wonderment is our emotional response as we witness the mysteries, the magic, and the beauty that genuinely surround us, especially when something transcends our current state of knowledge and comprehension. It is the catalyst of belief. The more we marvel at the complexities of life, the Universe, and all in between, the more meaning and truth we seek. Wonderment encourages us to receive the magic and wonder within the ordinary and the extraordinary.

Dr. Wayne Dyer says it beautifully: "Once you believe in yourself and see your soul as divine and precious, you will automatically be converted to a being that creates miracles." This is so beautifully spoken and so very true. It is something I have become witness to in every element of my life, and you will too. We are only as brilliant as the universal energy we allow to enter our lives, all ego, pride, fear, and doubt aside. We create these miracles by being open, trusting the process, and believing in everything yet to be known to us. If you could not achieve this for yourself, you would not be here reading this book. You can, and you will. I know this to be true for you. If you are drawn to or fear it, you must proceed forward consciously, bravely, boldly, and fearlessly in all that you set out to do, from healing to evolving to living a life fulfilled.

The archetype of your life as you know it is ready to reawaken and transcend, which is why this book arrived in your life when it did.

These are the moments that define lives, by choice. You are ready to make that choice. All you have to do is believe in all that you truly are. I believe in you, and I believe you are ready to make these beautiful choices for yourself too.

You are ready!

• • •

A defining moment for Olympic gold medal gymnast Mitch Gaylord when listening to his inner voice and believing in it wholeheartedly, for the first time but not the last, moved him in the direction of his dreams—helping the USA men's gymnastics team to win their first and only Olympic gold medal in the history of the sport, in the 1984 Olympic Games.

I am sharing this story with you because it shows how embracing the power of belief changed the course of Mitch's life and the course of Olympic history. Had Mitch not transcended his own fears and ego and believed that he could, he would not have, and many lives would have been different because of the choices he made on his journey that changed the history of the United States men's gymnastics team forever.

The power of belief is real, and you can live within it in every moment of your life, making every moment and dream come true for you and everyone who crosses your path.

The Big Decision

by Mitch Gaylord

In 1981, three years before the '84 Olympics, I found myself nowhere near where I wanted or needed to be in my gymnastics journey. I was hanging on to the seventh spot in the national rankings, and to add to that, I was designated as an alternate for the '81 world championship team. Mentally, physically, emotionally, I was in a bad place. Filled with self-doubt, frustration, and an overwhelming confusion about how to proceed, I was standing at a crossroads. One thing was clear: I needed a significant change that would reshape my destiny.

The catalyst for that transformation? It was an utterly magical twist of fate and a gut feeling more potent than anything I'd ever experienced.

Let me take you back to an unforgettable plane flight in 1981. I was flying home with my teammates from the '81 world championship in Moscow, Russia. Most of them were sound asleep, but I was wide-awake. The competition had been a disappointment. US men's gymnastics had faced a tough time, and to make matters worse, I was that guy on the sidelines, the alternate who never got the chance to prove himself.

Physically and mentally drained, I had just spent days in a foreign country watching the world's best gymnasts go head-to-head and questioning my fate. *When will I get my shot? Will I ever be one of the best? How on earth did I end up in this situation?*

That last question was the easiest to answer. You see, during the qualifying meet in the USA that determined the world championship team, I sprained my ankle while performing my floor routine. I admit it wasn't just that stumble that caused the setback. I hadn't performed up to par throughout the competition, making silly mistakes and failing to showcase my best self. And it was all in my head—I lacked belief in my abilities and the conviction that I belonged on that team.

The top six positions made up the team while the seventh, where I landed, was the dreaded alternate.

Back to that flight, where I was wallowing in depression, anger, and frustration, not just about the immediate situation but the prospect of returning home to a pretty dismal training environment. The coach I had at that time and I were not exactly the best of pals. It felt like he was trying to mold me into a clone of his pride and joy, Peter Vidmar, the country's top gymnast. I resisted fiercely, feeling like he was trying to shape me into something I was not.

Don't get me wrong, I held no grudges against Vidmar. He was a fantastic and exceptional gymnast, but we were worlds apart in personality and gymnastic style. Peter was the epitome of dedication and hard work, compensating for what I saw as a lack of natural talent with sheer effort, consistency, and determination. On the flip side, I had a bounty of raw talent but lacked the basics, discipline, and self-confidence.

I was confident I couldn't thrive under a coach who didn't believe in me in an environment where I felt like an outsider. But walking away from UCLA, despite the challenges, didn't seem like the right choice. After all, I was on a full scholarship at an exceptional institution. Where could I go? Who would coach me? What move could fix this mess?

So, as hard as I tried to shut down my mind during that seemingly endless flight, I couldn't. There were no solutions, no answers in sight. A sense of defeat engulfed me.

And then, out of nowhere, a tap on my shoulder jolted me from my thoughts. "Mitch, are you awake?" It was my idol, Kurt Thomas. He had left first class to find me and proposed a chat. He couldn't sleep either, he said, and he wanted to talk.

Honestly, I half thought I was dreaming. How was my idol, of all people, seeking out the alternate for a conversation? And not just any chat, but an invite to first class on a Boeing 747, the upstairs section that some might remember. I had barely exchanged a couple of sentences with Kurt before this. We'd crossed paths briefly at the 1980 Olympic trials, where I'd approached him excitedly, but he hadn't a clue who I was.

For those unfamiliar with Kurt Thomas, he reigned as our country's top gymnast for years. The World Champion in '79, he was our big hope for Olympic gold in 1980, a dream that got dashed when the US boycotted those Games. By 1981, he'd retired and was now in Moscow as ABC's expert commentator for the event.

So, I was sitting in first class on a 747 with the legendary Kurt Thomas. My heart raced, my palms sweated—it was a mix of disbelief and anxiety. Kurt began, "Mitch, can you open up about what's holding you back mentally from being the best gymnast in the country? You're the most talented, creative, and stylish gymnast, yet you don't see that in yourself. Unless you take the lead, our team won't improve beyond what we witnessed. I want to help you get there."

And that's how the conversation started. Kurt wanted to understand every facet of me—my childhood, my early days in gymnastics, and the present mess I was in. We talked for hours, and for the first time in my gymnastics journey, I felt heard, cared for, and believed in—more than I believed in myself.

I was convinced this encounter was fate, orchestrated by something beyond my understanding. As our conversation concluded, Kurt proposed to become my coach. He would train me daily, even as he embarked on a professional gymnastics tour in two months.

I knew it meant leaving behind my full-ride scholarship at UCLA, but my gut screamed that this was the way to my potential, the path to the pinnacle, the route to the '84 Olympics. Not a shred of doubt clouded my decision.

Upon returning home, things rapidly changed. Soon I was off to Florida to join Kurt's tour. Over the following months, I trained with Kurt relentlessly. When the tour started, we'd arrive in another city each day where we performed in front of live audiences. I learned the love of performing versus the fear of competition, which made all the difference in the world. I was no longer worried about the outcomes of completions, as I focused on performing to the best of my abilities and loving the process. After the performances and on our long bus rides between cities, we talked for hours, and each conversation fueled me with self-belief, guidance, and invaluable insights. It was with golden nuggets of self-talk, belief, and mindset.

Kurt's influence on my life and career was immeasurable, and I credit him and the choice to train under him for turning my career around. Here's what happened by following my gut, trusting in a higher power, and, most importantly, having the courage to act on it:

From seventh place in 1981 . . .

. . . to second place after six months of Kurt's training in 1982

. . . first place after my time with Kurt in 1983 (that's a tale for another day)

. . . first place again in 1984

. . . NCAA national champion

Then came the '84 Olympics—my teammates and I clinched its first-ever team gold, and I secured a silver in vaulting, along with bronze medals in rings and parallel bars.

Your Belief

*As you work through this book, have you begun to see
the patterns and beliefs that have brought you to this place in your life
where transformation could not be welcomed into your life?*

*Can you release your ego even more and embrace belief in
everything unknown to you now? Can you trust in your ability to allow
your soul, your intuition, to guide you through this transformation?
Can you believe that it will?*

*Can you see how the Universe has a plan much greater than
the one you set for yourself and trust in its power to bring it all to you
in divine timing by allowing it to unfold for you, as it has already begun?*

*Can you trust in the belief that you are already transforming and
opening up to who you truly are? Can you believe that feeling you have
carried with you all your life to now unfold for you in magical ways?*

Because it will and it is. **Meditation** *will light your way.*

Chapter Twelve

MEDITATION

Welcoming the Light Within

You must find the place within yourself where nothing is impossible.

— DEEPAK CHOPRA

Meditation is invaluable in our lives; it centers us and brings us back into balance. We live in such a fast-paced world, and meditation is one of the only ways to slow our lives down long enough to breathe and recapture our breath from the external world surrounding us.

In the rapid pace at which my life had always traveled, meditation was not something I believed I could ever do at all let alone successfully. Quieting my inner critiques, dialogues, and distractions was far too difficult for me, as my state of consciousness had not allowed me to sit in stillness or silence long enough to achieve a quiet and peaceful balance in between worlds.

That changed when I reached a certain level of healing where I was able to become still and silent and surrender. Being able to surrender myself and commit to doing my inner work gave me a much deeper appreciation and understanding of meditation, its endless benefits, and the many ways of consistently achieving this state of being within my life, not just while practicing meditation but within every moment of my life.

My Journey into Meditation

Meditation captured my attention many times throughout my life. I was guided toward it in many different ways until I integrated it into my daily rituals much later in life. Before then, I was fearful of it, to be completely honest. I feared what I might find in the silence of meditation, how I would hear the messages and the guidance I would receive (if any), how I might interpret the messages I would receive, or that I would find a more profound void than the one I had known before. All these fear-based feelings and emotions haunted me for decades until I finally succumbed and discovered the magic that is meditation.

I was first introduced to meditation through Deepak Chopra, M.D., over 24 years ago while working in corporate America. The introduction to Deepak himself and his work was fascinating, and I was fascinated by him. He was intelligent, he was authentic, and he was a genuine advocate of this philosophy. During my spare time, which was minimal back then, I would read, and his books became part of my repertoire of must-reads. I was astounded by his quest and passion to transition from conventional medicine to a more alternative and holistic approach to health and wellness. I was also amazed to learn that he, too, believed that traditional medicine had its limitations. I had always felt this was true and believed the mind-body connection was the most profound, especially regarding mind-body medicine and healing. At the time, I had no idea how impactful this would become in my life. I knew that the mind-body connection existed, and I was fascinated by it. Now I understand why I was fascinated by the mind-body connection, as it did become a monumental part of my journey, my purpose, my passion, and my healing years later when I finally put it into practice.

In my many efforts to embody a meditation practice, I searched for greater meaning and knowledge via the most widely known leaders in meditation, from Deepak Chopra to Paramahansa Yogananda, the Dalai Lama, Thich Nhat Hanh, Eckhart Tolle, and many others. I dove deep into their philosophies and teachings. I even completed a course with Deepak Chopra and Roger Gabriel. I was so drawn to meditation, but not in the conventional way. I wanted to learn, and I wanted to go deeper. I wanted to find that place deep within that meditation takes you to. I wanted to live there, within its light, and I made every valiant effort to do so.

After many unsuccessful attempts, I finally achieved this state of being in my meditations. Once I did, I would come out of my meditation, embracing this light within, and then try to maintain this state throughout each moment of my day. I did not want to experience this only while in meditation; I wanted this light with me always, as I knew it was an essential part of living a more conscious and meaningful life. This was when meditation became an essential part of my journey, and I committed to it each and every day. It was this profound light connecting my heart and soul to something so much greater than myself that embraced me in absolute enlightenment. It was a feeling of light that emanated throughout my body. Everything sparkled, from my toes to my crown—a feeling you will feel, too, once you let go.

When I first began to take this feeling from meditation with me throughout my day, I was determined to hold on to it no matter what life offered me. I focused on feeling the light, the peace, and the connection I felt throughout my day. It was the difference between living a conscious life versus an unconscious one, and I knew it. This light within is so bright, beautiful, and brilliant that once you feel it, you will want to live within it and not without it. It is breathtaking, and it is magical, as you will soon see and acknowledge it for yourself.

Meditation through Enduring Challenges

Life was constantly challenging me throughout my healing journey and trying its best to wake me up to my truth. The challenges kept coming with a much greater force each time until I did. Before doing this body of work and achieving this level of consciousness through implementing it, and incorporating meditation, I would choose to shut down and move through the challenges without emotion as a shell of a person. After experiencing this level of consciousness, challenges began to affect me differently, unlike they once had. They were not at all debilitating as they once were to me. This work and meditation opened me up even more to this new reality and perspective on each situation I was in or could look back upon now. I realized that these circumstances were all trying to teach me something invaluable and something I desperately needed to learn in this lifetime.

I found that I was consciously beginning to let go of all that no longer served my life and all that was holding me back from living the life I truly desired without hesitation, doubt, fear, or pain. I was now deeply connected to this light energy guiding me like nothing I had ever known before, and I trusted it every step of the way. I was centered within it, and I was listening to it. It opened up the gateway to my intuition, which was now fully supported. I now knew what to do and no longer feared doing it. This state of consciousness was free from the many barriers I myself had built. I could follow my truth as it appeared to me with each breath and in everything I did. I was being guided, and I knew it. Staying centered, open, and in this conscious way of being was now my intention as it brought everything together for me and will for you too.

There were some days when I could not find the time to meditate, so I began learning how to connect within this level of consciousness that made everything in my life flow. It is where I began to explore other ways to connect and stay connected. I started by observing everything in my daily life where I could find a sense of balance or reprieve, and this is when I had another epiphany. As you begin to live more consciously, epiphanies will become a daily occurrence *(smiling)*. It was through finding ways of living consciously within the things I loved to do that I incorporated meditation into my daily life, no matter what I faced. This is what allowed me to stay connected no matter the circumstances. It allowed me to find peace, which meant eliminating all that did not bring me peace. Meditation will bring you even more clarity as you begin to implement this work into your own life. You will begin to see the pieces that were once shattered fall back into place more profoundly and beautifully as you become stronger with each day.

Finding Meditation through Movement

For me, meditation involved intentional movement: classical Pilates, yoga, tai chi, qigong, walking in nature, swimming, mindful stretching, dancing, running, and jogging. When I engage in movements like these, I flow through each movement mindfully while concentrating on the sensations in my body, my breathing, and being present. It is very calming to me. When I am doing tai chi and qigong, the movements are smooth and graceful, and they emphasize mindfulness and relaxation, allowing me to be fully present in my body. Swimming is another one. I love the feeling of the water on my skin as I move through it. I connect with my strokes, movement, and rhythm as I swim. I love to run and jog because I love the feeling of forward motion and can connect easily to that feeling. It is easy to immerse yourself in being present while running or jogging because you focus on being present in the moment without distractions or you might fall, like I do sometimes *(smiling)*. It all keeps you connected to your body, just like meditation does so beautifully.

Mindful stretching is a great way to connect with your breath and body. It is a gentle way to wake up and go to bed. Dancing is also wonderful because you can feel the rhythm and the vibration of the music within every ounce of your being. It is inspiring and invigorating for the soul.

Finding meditation through movement has been life-changing for me. It is a wonderful way to intertwine mindfulness, intentional actions, and physical activity while nurturing a more profound connection within your body, mind, and soul. I do many of these things in the privacy of my home or at studios that I trust to ensure the right environment, as your surroundings will support you in being present and connected, which is vital.

These are all ways to support you in living consciously throughout your day, as they keep you connected to that beautiful light within that this work and meditation connect you to.

Practicing Meditation

When I practice my meditations at home, I always ensure that I create a peaceful environment for myself and my family if they join me, whether they practice with me or near me. Family meditations are quite beautiful, and if there are children in your home, they will benefit from them in many beautiful ways.

I start by creating a calm and peaceful place where I will not be disturbed. This allows me to relax, knowing I will not be interrupted by anything other than my mind *(smiling)*. It also helps calm my nervous system, a vital benefit of meditation.

After I get comfortable, I begin by practicing deep breathing. I focus on my breath entering my body and leaving my body. I visualize it as a white light that sparkles, moving through me. It centers me and focuses me inward. Sometimes I use ambient music or guided meditations using an app such as Calm, but silence is always best. Silence puts you in a much deeper state of relaxation in your mind, body, and soul.

Once in this state of relaxation, I focus on my body from my toes to my crown, tuning in to where I might be holding on to any tensions or stressors. I then consciously release them in those areas.

Once I have released my body from any pressures or stressors, I begin to visualize that I am in a tranquil, beautiful, and peaceful place I love. In this quiet place, I become even calmer. If my mind wanders, as it tends to, I focus on breathing while asking myself questions. The following questions are a great way to begin. I learned them during my studies with Deepak Chopra and Roger Gabriel. The questions are: *Who am I? What do I want? What am I grateful for? What is my purpose?* You can ask yourself any questions you would like answers to. Questions are a direct pathway to going even deeper within. Your soul's purpose is revealed as you evolve in this place.

Then, when my mind becomes peaceful and centered again, I can refocus on any sensations I feel within and throughout my body, as this always helps guide me inward. The most important element of meditation is being patient. It is a practice, and like all things practiced, it takes time to master. But once you master it (and you will), you will be forever grateful for it and to it, as it will change your life in extraordinary and beautiful ways.

Meditation has had an extraordinary effect on me and my life. This did not happen quickly, but gradually, and more and more as I made space for meditation and allowed it to take me where I needed to go. It would have happened much sooner had I been more open to it, but I relentlessly fought it to hold on to any control I believed I still had over my life. Control is a delusion, an illusion we create in times of fear. It is something that you will effortlessly learn to let go of, as it indeed does not exist.

As you make space for meditation, you will experience a new-found sense of balance and centeredness. The unceasing noise of the world surrounding you will become quieter, and the symphony of your thoughts will become harmonious. Stress, anxiety, and worry will begin to release their grip on you, as they will no longer be reliable companions. You will find yourself in the calm of your life with a sense of peace that will stay with you beyond the moments of meditation. The calm and peace will flow into every moment of your life. It took time for me to master this level of consciousness, but once I did, I learned how to embrace it and then hold on to it and take it with me throughout my life. Once you feel it, you will know how important it is and will be to you and your life. Once you feel this light, you can carry it with you throughout your life as you embrace it more and more. It will become very natural to you and for you to do.

During my meditations, I realized what guided me toward meditation was not only the profound fascination it held for me but its power to create a sacred space for me to be in the present, where I could then remain within its light. This state of being is essential as our world pulls at us endlessly and in countless ways that demand our full attention and scatter us away from our truth and inner light. In meditation, and within its sanctuary, time slows down and stands still, creating the pathway to our inner essence.

The significance of this practice in your life will become clearer to you as you navigate through life's challenges with a newfound purpose, passion, grace, and a deeper appreciation and understanding of your circumstances and the lessons in which they came into your life to teach you. You will also learn to free yourself from your ego's limitations, which will do wonders for your mental, emotional, spiritual, and physical wellness. Releasing your ego will unbind you from the thoughts, emotions, and stories that you tell yourself about yourself, which are not your truth or in your best interest to hold on to. This work and meditation will set you free from these limitations as you realize that who you truly are is not based within your thoughts but in your heart and soul, your truth.

Meditation is one of the most profound practices of awakening and reawakening to your soul's essence and purpose. It is invaluable to you and your journey. As you engage with it, you will not be overpowered by fear, guilt, or pain any longer. You will embrace the ancient wisdom within you and feel safe within the silence of your truth.

Meditation is the most compassionate form of intimacy with oneself. Your truth and ability to go deep within you and connect with your soul's magic are you at your very essence. This light will show you just how beautiful you truly are, in all ways.

Find a place in your life to begin practicing meditation if you have not already. Learn to become still, even for a few minutes a day, as it is an essential way to begin that will support you in balancing and centering yourself, leaving you calm and at peace to see with such clarity. Once you achieve this state, you will not wish to live without it, and you will learn with time how to maintain it throughout every minute of your life and journey. Embrace it and connect with it as it is magical; in essence, it is your truth. It is ALL YOU.

Introducing Randi Marks

At the beginning of my healing journey, I worked with an incredible teacher named Randi Marks. She saw things in me that I was not ready to see at first. She was patient and nurturing in such a way that I could not deny her words, as she always spoke her own truth and her truth of *me*. She is a healer, and she supported the healer in me. For this book, I asked her to write about meditation and what it means to her, as she and I are very much alike in our quest to help people heal their bodies. I asked her to share with you the practices that help her embrace a meditative state. I did not prep her by telling her specifically what I was writing about in this chapter; I wanted to see how aligned we were in our thinking—and we are.

As you heal and evolve, people will either evolve with you or out of your life. The good ones stay with you always. Randi was one of them for me.

Opening Ourselves to the Spiritual World

BY RANDI MARKS

Which voice will you listen to?

A battle exists between our soul and our inner critic (the voice of the Opponent)—which tricks us through our egos, attachments, fears, and limited beliefs. Meditation becomes a powerful tool to overcome these addictions and gives us the energy to seek peace and harmony. You win the battle by recognizing that your inner critic, feelings, and reactions are illusionary. The fact that you see and feel this internal fight is an excellent first step in knowing that these internal forces exist.

The challenge is overcoming our familiarity with our ego, which is comfortable and becomes who we are. Meditation helps us transcend the ego and amplify the energy of our soul. It is part of our spiritual journey that we came here to gradually transform both the body and mind's instincts to follow the soul.

Energetically, meditation reveals our reactivity. Through the breath, we draw in light to illuminate our darkness; we birth a new Soul through new consciousness. Our work is to create a vessel that can contain this light. If we cannot do so, that light cannot reveal itself. This is why meditation must become a consistent practice.

We constantly expand our vessels and awaken through reflection, inquiry, or meaningful conversations. Technology and social media have bombarded us with the Opponent's energy, and we must replace that negativity with constant wisdom, a supportive environment, and power that elevates the volume of the Soul.

People feel they lack control over their destiny. Meditation changes that.

Creating a daily practice puts your life's power back into your hands. It becomes a sacred time where you step out of the chaos and move into higher dimensions, which are feelings of total peace. With every breath, the life force moves through you, providing reassurance that everything will be okay.

We need more than saying we want to change. We must get to the spiritual source of why we behaved that way in the first place, remove the source of reactivity from our consciousness, and diminish its power over us. Each day, before you meditate, ask to be shown what is causing a disturbance inside of you. Where did it come from? How can you lessen its effect on your consciousness? Where do emotions manifest in your body? Does it also show up in your health? Then, spend time with your eyes closed, following your breath, and listening. Trust the messages you receive. Remove doubt and replace it with certainty that everything comes from the light, including the answers.

All the negativity, challenges, doubts, and fears are sent to us to bring the growth we need. Each of us has aspects of our soul that need correcting. The negativity we label bad pushes the Creator's Light into our lives. The Creator sees what He needs to do for us, determines the level of consciousness we need, and creates that situation for us. A person goes through challenges and, from those challenges, perfects their soul in an exact way.

Three common excuses why people don't meditate are:

- I do not have time.
- I am doing it wrong.
- I have too many thoughts.

You have time, there is no wrong way to meditate, and you will have thoughts the entire time you meditate. The mind has more than 70,000 thoughts a day. It is up to you, each of us, to decide whether we want to be aware of those thoughts. If we do not face them, they get pushed down into our subconscious mind, determining our reality. If you are unhappy with your life, getting intimate with your thoughts is the best way to change that. Your life transforms when you become aware and shift your old thoughts to newer, more empowering ones. To control your destiny is to be in power of your conscious mind.

As you advance in your practice, you will notice the internal chatter quieting, making it easier to enter into a state of oneness. Use your breath to shift your focus from a thought to a breath. Like a wave in the ocean, you will notice the views pulling you out and the breath pulling you back in. Go with the flow and ride the wave. Soon enough, the thoughts will cease. This process begins to retrain the mind that it is not in control. You are. It becomes a compelling lesson for any meditator, spilling over into all aspects of your life.

I wake up each day knowing that today is all that matters. If you can prepare your consciousness first thing in the morning to prepare yourself for the challenges that will arise throughout the day that will transform the past and create blessings for the future.

If you have difficulty sitting still, walk in nature, go for a run, dance to music, or write out your thoughts and create goals. Do whatever you can to ground your energy, find peace within, and process the unfavorable mental chatter. We must learn to find calm in the chaos of our busy lives. We achieve this by retreating into ourselves for a few minutes each day.

Here is an example of what my daily practice looks like:

Every morning, I take an audit of my life by checking in with how I am feeling. I look at my emotions, challenges, or any lack. I ask myself how I feel physically, mentally, emotionally, and spiritually. I ask to be shown moments of pain and disconnection and invite the light to show me what issue to pay attention to within this situation. If I feel pain or tension, I send my intention and breath there until I feel it lessen. Then I bring my attention back to my entire body and center myself. I continue breathing with my eyes closed until I feel complete and peaceful. Lastly, I acknowledge the answers I received and thank the Creator for returning my soul to my body and allowing me to live another day.

Here are some concepts to help you start your meditation practice, but know the list is endless. Get creative and enjoy the process! Meditate on:

- The Light around you
- A question or situation
- Your health
- Angels
- Your Soul
- A loved one
- Your desires
- An action to take
- The emptying of your mind
- An emotional struggle
- A word, affirmation, or sound
- An emotion you struggle with

As I write about meditation, I am hoping that you find the space in your life for meditation along this transformational journey. It will support you in so many profound and beautiful ways. Your life is changing, and meditation will help to light the way.

Your Meditation

Can you make space in your life for meditation? Can you open yourself up to its many benefits and allow it to guide you even more in partnership with your intuition and the Universe surrounding you?

Are you willing to let go enough to allow meditation to shed light on your life's circumstances and guide you toward your soul's purpose?

Can you allow yourself to live consciously every day and with every breath? Can you embrace the light of meditation and the light in all you do and want to do in your life?

Can you be guided away from all that no longer serves your life and purpose? Can you release these people and circumstances with love, understanding, and compassion for you and them?

Will you begin practicing meditation today?

Meditation supports us in connecting us to all things, and **connection** *is essential in all things.*

Chapter Thirteen

CONNECTION

Experiencing Oneness and Togetherness

One can have no smaller or greater mastery than mastery of oneself.

— LEONARDO DA VINCI

Living consciously is the beauty that connection to yourself brings you. Mastering connection is something we are all born with the ability to do and something that will profoundly evolve our lives in the most beautiful ways. Connection to yourself and to all things will be, by far, your most significant achievement in this lifetime and something that you will cherish as your life takes on a whole new meaning. It is where your transformation comes to fruition in more ways than you can imagine.

The undeniable truth about connection is that we cannot feel it with anyone or anything until we feel it within ourselves. Connection is the most intimate way of life and form of communication that we can have with ourselves and then share with others. All relationships should be intimate ones. Surround yourself with others with whom you can share yourself deeply without hiding any element of who you genuinely are in your very essence. There are so many beautiful ways to find intimacy in life, but connecting within yourself and with others in a more meaningful way is, by far, its purest and most sacred form.

Living in the Darkness of Unconsciousness

In the world that we live in, disconnecting and disassociating have become commonplace, almost expected, unfortunately to a fault. This has created a tremendous void within our lives. By allowing ourselves to live within this void, we gravitate toward people, places, and things that we would not have had we been connected within our own energy force, our soul. It derails us from our soul's purpose and deprives us of the lives we came here to live and thrive within. You are already aware of this and can feel it deep within you. It has become far too easy for us to shut down and stop communicating in the way we truly wish to and are meant to, which brings us heartache, sorrow, and loneliness, a feeling that we cannot shake until we are ready to. These moments of denial, regret, and resentment grow within us, leaving us unmoving and in the void rather than experiencing a more fulfilling life. Joy, happiness, and bliss cannot live in this disconnection from the soul; nothing real can.

Connection to all things is where the real magic is, and by magic, I am not speaking of anything foo-foo or fluffy. I am talking about walking in the wake of the life you came here to create and will create for yourself. I'm talking about acknowledging the lives you directly and indirectly affect—since every choice you make, consciously or unconsciously, affects another person, perhaps more than one person, as it affects you.

If you are living unconsciously, those choices will negatively affect you and others, leading to more trauma that you will carry within your body.

Living in the Light of Consciousness

In living consciously, every choice you make in faith will amaze and awaken you. It is where the magic is—walking within your oneness and in truth with who you are without hiding behind anything, including your work. It has become the staple of long-lived excuses and facades that people still use today to hide behind. If you make yourself too busy to connect with who you are, you are living in the shadows of your life and not the light of your life. I know this because I was one of those people. Looking back now, it feels as if I was living in between two separate worlds (unconscious and conscious). Now those two worlds are worlds apart, and I am living in oneness, present and conscious. It is not in your best interest to continue to play small, as the unconscious mind is just that—playing small by abiding by fear rather than the courage you have within you to do all that you are pulled and drawn to do. This is not who you are. If you were not ready to make this move, you would not be reading this book. You are more spiritually aware now than ever. There is something much greater at work here for you, and it awaits you and your life. You are ready to step forward and own it. It is your soul's purpose. It is why you are here reading this book, as you have quite a large purpose to fulfill. Your body brought you to this place so that you could awaken or reawaken to your truth. It did not do this to hurt you or punish you; it simply needed to find a way through to you so that you can find a way through to others, including yourself, first and foremost. You have a powerful purpose, and it is time to own it and take your power back by empowering yourself to move toward your hopes and dreams, as only you can bring them to life in your own special and unique way.

Connection is the only way forward. I know that you have had moments when you felt connected and felt its magic. The light radiated within you in those moments. You can embrace your light with every ounce of your being and shine it upon this world uniquely. Being connected and staying connected is you in your most powerful form. "Powerful" meaning walking within the path of your soul's purpose, and you know what that is for you or you will very soon. If it feels big, it is because it is big and extraordinarily significant. If we all walked in our light, consciously and connected, our world would change, and it needs to. For centuries, we have conformed to believe that which others wish us to when, in essence, all you have ever needed to know and understand is already within you. Connecting to that essence will change everything for you; it will give you your life back. No one or thing will ever be able to take that away from you again as it is yours, and only you know what that gift is for you.

You will be astonished at how quickly your life will change once you connect with this essence, light, within you and surrender to it fully. Miracles will unfold right before your eyes in ways you could not have imagined or created for yourself while living in the void of your unconscious mind. It will be captivating and unexplainable but something you will cherish and hold on to as you live out the rest of your life, witnessing it all unfold before you. It will shift you into living a more conscious life, as you will not wish to live within the shadows of your life ever again once you reach this point of reawakening, and you will. You already know that this is what you want, so fighting it is like fighting yourself, and we have all done enough of that *(smiling)*. It is time to evolve into who you authentically are and get ready to glow!

If you could not shine your brightness and brilliance in this world and this lifetime, you would not be where you are right now, reading this book.

Shining brilliantly is your birthright. You were born for something so much more significant than the life that you have chosen and are currently living. It is time to embrace who you are in your essence and open yourself up to the infinite possibilities that await you. Connecting to your light and staying connected to it throughout everything life brings forth, including the tests and tribulations that have come and will come to strengthen you and keep you committed to your journey. It is your way forward. The tests will feel lighter and lighter the more conscious you become. Commit to yourself, commit to your healing, and commit to living the life you came here to live and not the life your unconscious self-created for you, as it no longer serves you. You can safely close that chapter and leave it behind you now. Be grateful to and for it, but know that you have officially outgrown and evolved from underneath it because you have.

There are many ways to connect and stay connected. The most important way is by doing this inner work and connecting to your soul, light, higher self, heart chakra, solar plexus, or source. It is within your energy force, your life force, where you will begin to live your most extraordinary and exceptional life with peace, harmony, and balance guiding you. It is where you will find harmony and balance in your life and where your life will unfold in profound and miraculous ways.

Becoming self-aware will become natural as you understand your thoughts and desires more deeply. You will begin to understand the choices that brought you to this place and why you made them. This is where forgiveness comes in—forgiving yourself for the past and releasing yourself from it. You cannot take it with you, and you do not want to. Living within the restraints and regrets of the past will only continue to hold you back and suffocate you. It all happened to awaken you or reawaken you, so to speak, to your soul's purpose.

When connected, you will see, feel, and understand the fears that have held you back, and you will release them because they will take on a whole new meaning—one that connects you with all that you have been through and then sheds light on who you have become as a result of having these experiences.

When you are connected, fear cannot penetrate you, as your light will guide you forward and protect you in a way that makes you feel safe within your life and body. You will feel more emotionally sound as you manage your emotions more effectively. You will be able to recognize them and honor them without being controlled by them. You will become emotionally resilient as you see them for what they are and move through them quickly rather than allowing them to linger on. You will become more disciplined and be able to stay on course without allowing temptation or distractions to derail you from achieving your soul's purpose. You will remain committed to your desires and make choices that will make YOU happy, which will have a very positive effect on your life rather than a negative one. Your purpose will become apparent to you, and you will be able to work patiently toward it and achieve it with grace and a newfound determination that you will have complete faith in as you will know and feel it to be true for you.

With each day, you will witness your growth and development, both personal and professional, with fresh, new eyes. You will be more willing to learn from your experiences in a way that uplifts you versus bringing you pain, sorrow, or sadness. You will begin to expand in every way imaginable and unimaginable by empowering and allowing yourself to do so. You will openly be willing to release and allow the Universe to create magic in your life because you know it will. You will feel calm and at peace, enabling you to make choices with intention, mindfulness, and patience while avoiding impulsive actions of the past that may lead to undesirable consequences, granting you even more power and awareness over your emotions.

You will feel more empowered. The more connected you are to your soul and body, the more connected you become. Practicing this kind of mindfulness, presence, and connection with each moment of your life will become so natural that you will not even notice your effort, as it will become effortless. You will not react in the ways that you once did. Triggers will no longer trigger you, as you will see beyond all of it. It will also allow you the freedom from judgment of yourself and others because you will come to understand that we all have our journeys to navigate through. We all come here with challenges that we must learn and overcome in this lifetime to evolve into our most significant selves and live our most fulfilling lives. It is there for every one of us.

When challenges and setbacks do arise, you will become more emotionally and psychologically resilient to them. You will be better able to bounce back completely and in a fraction of the time it took before, with a more positive attitude, a confident presence, and a solid sense of self and inner strength, as you will know, and believe, that you can and will navigate through it effortlessly.

You will find realignment by self-reflecting and reevaluating your life by observing when you aligned with your heart's desires and soul's purpose, and you knew it, only, you denied it at the time. It will open you up even more to living in alignment with your heart, mind, soul, and body in the presence of your life, which will ensure forward movement and momentum.

Living consciously fills your soul with empathy and compassion for all things, especially yourself. Relationships will become more evident to you, and you will be able to relate with others on a much deeper emotional level as you will understand that their actions reflect where they are on their journey and not a reflection of you. You will see how interacting with certain people has helped you to evolve and has helped them grow in ways that perhaps you were both meant to. When you can look at all the relationships in your life with empathy and compassion, you will release the pain of holding on to them, allowing you to forgive and let go more quickly if necessary, and you will know when it is. In most cases, it was most likely long overdue. There is great power and strength in this place of release and forgiveness. There is no greater connection in this Universe than to the oneness you feel within yourself, as, in this energy force, you connect to the infinite, which is boundless.

Being connected within these depths of your soul is the most profound connection to self that you will ever experience. It is your authentic, spiritual, and emotional well-being, wrapped up in this beautiful and divine embodiment of oneness, that you will feel with every ounce of your being. It transcends all superficial thoughts and emotions. They do not exist in this energy. This interconnectedness and inner knowingness is your energy force and intuition waiting and wanting to guide you. By being in this state of connected consciousness, you are opening yourself up to truly listen, feel, and be guided by this phenomenal force that will light the way for you. It will bring you all you desire in perfect and divine timing. And when the timing comes, you will see the divinity in it. I never thought I would, and I did. It not only happened in perfect timing, but it happened with absolute perfection, as in when I was ready enough to receive it without sabotaging it. Trust the process, and you will prosper in so many beautiful ways. It will leave you speechless at times, as it did for me. People who know me know that I am not ever at a loss for words *(smiling)*.

The ways in which your life will evolve and change are limitless. As you align with who you are, you will see how your desires and needs will evolve as you do. Your limiting beliefs will vanish from your thoughts as you realize just how limitless and boundless you genuinely are, and the opportunities will soon follow, providing you with undeniable confirmation. You will see them as the miracles they are. Your connections with people will also evolve as you do. Once you reach this level of enlightenment, you will find that people who are not ready or even willing to meet you where you are and who are not continuing to evolve as you do will soon depart from your life. It may be painful in some relationships, but you will soon realize it is in your best interest and theirs to release them and let them go. If people do not align with your evolution and do not support your continued growth and enlightenment, they will consciously or unconsciously try to hold you back. It only hurts you because relationships like these do not flourish like you may have hoped they would. They are only catalysts in your transformation and evolution. With time, you will be grateful for them, as they were essential pieces of those lovely life lessons that will continue to show up until we wake up *(smiling)*.

Connections of the Heart

Some of the most painful life lessons are those of the heart, and soul connections are no different. When we are disconnected from our light, we tend to attract others into our lives who are equally disconnected, or more so. Some are even entirely damaged. In these relationships, you will try to focus on their healing over your own, but that only ends in a much more significant loss for you as you will lose yourself within those relationships, and your healing will cease to exist. You may perceive these relationships as love, but you are settling for less than what you truly deserve and desire out of fear, loneliness, and self-doubt. When you begin to do this work, you will realize that the healing starts within you, first and foremost. All healing begins within the connection to your energy force, your life force, your inner self, and your light. You cannot find it in another, nor can you heal another.

Once you enter this beautiful and sacred space, you will begin to attract healthier relationships with people who are committed to their healing and who will share in your completeness because they, too, will be complete within themselves, their healing, and oneness. This is very important, as it is when you will experience love in all of its beauty, love that is passionate, compassionate, truthful, kind, thoughtful, mindful, supportive, and filled with joy, happiness, bliss, and intimate moments that will feel like nothing you have ever experienced before. It will be a love built on friendship, honor, respect, and mutual adoration. Healthy in all ways, especially regarding communication and connection that will form its foundation.

There will be no guessing games, no mind games, no ghosting, no gaslighting, no disappearing acts, no narcissistic or abusive behaviors, and no self-serving behaviors, as you will find these character traits unacceptable because they are unacceptable. You will stop attracting any of them into your life because you will understand that these traits in others are unhealthy, and you will not wish to partake in the drama, chaos, and dysfunction that come with these traits.

I was never one to tolerate any of these behaviors, but I did once, and I will never allow it in my life again. People who treat people in these ways are beyond selfish and self-serving. It is best to RUN at the first sign of any of these traits than to stay, as no one with such qualities is worth your peace, especially when you are healing. These types of people are often damaged, so damaging you will feel natural to them—so distance yourself from them at the first sign. You do not need to engage negatively with them; walk away peacefully. As you become more and more enlightened, you will see the signs within minutes of meeting someone like this. You will sense it. Something will feel off or not right about them, or you may even pick up an energy that feels dark. Energy does not deceive. If it feels dark, it is dark. Always go with your first gut instinct, or intuition, on this. It is never wrong.

Connections We Are Born With

Family is another element of human and soulful connection that connects us to ourselves in ways that can root us either in fear or in love. For some, family is a beautiful gathering of people who genuinely love one another unconditionally while providing understanding, empathy, support, safety, and protection to grow, evolve, and flourish spiritually into who you are. For these people, family offers a secure foundation and the tools to thrive and navigate life's challenges.

For others, family is a source of dysfunction, chaos, and drama where you grow up with undiagnosed trauma buried deeply within each cell of your body. If that is not enough, abandonment, detachment, and emotional issues will negatively impact your life until you reach the point where you know you need to create a significant shift. You will feel like you might not escape it, but you will.

Every situation is so very different, yet every situation offers incredible life lessons. As you do this work, your connection to your current family may strengthen and deepen, or you may find what I call your soul family. Whether you grew up in a safe home environment or one that was not so safe for you to be who you truly are, you will get to this place where you will be guided toward those who will offer you the love and support you are meant to receive.

Family can create expectations for us that are not true to who we are on a soul level and may not coincide with what we feel our soul's purpose is. This can cause inner conflict, but as you connect with who you are in essence, these conflicts will also disappear. You will know what you have to do for the life that you wish to live, and you will follow through with it on your terms, as there is no other way for you once you reach this kind of clarity.

Your family members will either rise to the occasion to support you in your journey or distance themselves from you. Either way, you must live true to who you are and your purpose in this life, as this will bring you your most fulfilling and meaningful life. As you evolve, you will start to attract your soul family. They may not be biologically related to you, but they are spiritually there for you in the ways that matter the most. These people will support you in all the ways that will impact your life and healing in a genuine way, and you will do the same for them. These are the people who can see it for themselves and can see it for you and will want you to have it. They will hold space for you to grow and evolve, encouraging and inspiring you along your journey. They will vastly differ from those who will end up departing your life, as those individuals could not see it for themselves, so they could not see it for you and did not want you to have it. You will feel at home with your soul family in ways you might not have with your biological family. These are all connections you were born with just the same.

It is not a selfish act for you to make choices like these that support you on your journey. It is essential. It is your life, and you get to live it boundlessly. You deserve to surround yourself with people who are equally connected to who they are so that they can connect with you in more meaningful ways and vice versa. We have all lost so much by giving ourselves away to people who were not worthy of all we gave them. But these people taught us a great deal about ourselves, so be grateful for them in that way and move on from them with good intentions.

Your soul family will feel like individuals with whom you have a profound spiritual or soul connection that goes beyond biological family ties. You will have a deep sense of recognition, familiarity, and home when you meet them. They will share very similar core values and a sense of purpose with you. They will be drawn to similar life paths, inspirations, interests, and causes and will work with you to achieve these shared and individual goals that you will share with them and have for yourself. They will have an unwavering love for you and you for them. They will support and accept you for who you are and your choice to live your desired life. You will grow, evolve, and continue to evolve spiritually together. It will feel like home, and they will feel like family to you and you to them. It truly is beautiful to experience, and you will experience this if you have not already. They come in many different forms.

If you have children, you will feel more connected to them and more in love with them as you will begin to see them for their uniqueness and be able to support them in a way that helps them on their journey. You will be a role model to everyone in your life, and your children will benefit most from this as your healing will teach them how to live their lives to the fullest as you will inspire them in new and profound ways. I have seen it in my children. They know how to meditate and connect and are learning to live in that space. Watching them evolve in these ways has been breathtaking. Giving this to them now, or at any age, is one of the greatest gifts you can give your children other than the gift of life itself. Your connection to them will evolve and develop as they do. It will inspire you and your children and everyone who surrounds you.

Communication and Connection

Communication is another area that improves when you connect with your inner light. Communication has gone astray since text messaging and social media have entered our lives. Though those means of communicating hold value, they simply are not enough when it comes to genuine connection. A healthy and successful relationship with anyone is impossible if your relationship relies entirely on text messaging and e-mail. To feel a real connection with someone in a memorable and meaningful way that has depth, passion, compassion, and love, you have to be able to truly communicate, which means speaking to each other and sharing time and hearing each other's voices so that you can clearly connect with your feelings and their feelings, emotions, and most importantly, their words and how they express themselves. Energy is what we connect with, and platforms like text messaging and e-mail are devoid of energy—all the energy gets lost in translation. Connect with people personally, profoundly, intimately, and soulfully so that all relationships will become more meaningful to you and them.

Community and Connection

Community is another beautiful way to connect in even more ways that support our growth. Whether we build a community of our own in business or our personal lives, live in a community that we love, or participate in a support group or local community events, we connect in meaningful ways that support our lives and the lives of others. They not only nurture us in togetherness, but they remove us from isolation, and that does wonders for our souls. They give us a sense of joy, excitement, and even healing. Living in a community you love and an environment you love is essential for your soul. If where you live does not inspire you, and you can no longer connect with it, it is time to move on from there and find a home that speaks to you and your soul. Your soul will take you there. If you are drawn to a place, intrigued by a place, or curious about a place, start there first, as that is calling for you. Every place that drew me to it that I lived in or visited was some of my life's best and most magical moments and memories.

Being connected to your soul offers you such clarity in your life. It truly changes everything, and quite quickly, too. For me, it was instantaneous. When you feel something is true for you, it turns out to be true and unfolds right before you. If you did not believe in miracles before, you will soon or again, as that is how powerful and miraculous being connected and living a consciously connected life is. There is nothing more pure or true.

Healing and Connection

When it comes to healing your body, once you are connected and in oneness with your heart, mind, soul, and body, your body will speak to you in ways that will allow it to heal itself. You will know what to nourish your body with and when to. Your body will guide you toward the foods it needs to heal in unexplainable ways. It may come to you in your thoughts, in visions, or you may crave it. Either way, it comes through to you; listen to it. It is a sense that can be felt in many ways. When you pick something up or hold something in your hand, you will sense that your body is saying yes to it or no to it. If you proceed with a food or supplement that your body has not responded well to, you will feel uncomfortable, experiencing bloating, stomach aches, digestive issues, stiffness, and insomnia, to name a few. Your body will also make you more aware of what you put into your body that contributes to your illness and the symptoms you are experiencing. You will be so in tune with every ounce of your body that healing can profoundly occur. Food is vital in this way, and being connected to your body is one of the more profound ways to heal your body.

Healthy Boundaries

Healthy boundaries are essential in honoring your healing, your journey, and your connection to your inner light. Boundaries celebrate who you once were and who you have become and are becoming. You can permit yourself to have healthy boundaries and hold to them as they will distinguish themselves between surviving and thriving in health and healing. Healthy boundaries help you preserve your peace and protect you from the individuals, feelings, and emotions that have disturbed and disrupted your peace. It is like surrounding yourself with a bright white light or a sparkly bubble that keeps you connected to who you are and does not allow things that try to burst your bubble or put out your light close enough to you for that to happen. Making peace with the past and stepping into the present moment free from the burdens you once carried and took on as your own is healthy. We have all taken on burdens, so releasing them, connecting to who you are in your essence, and moving forward boundlessly in that connection will pave a new pathway for you free from the turbulence of the past. You have held yourself accountable long enough. It is safe to forgive, ask for forgiveness, give yourself closure, and move on in this new and vibrant direction.

By healing your body and connecting within your inner light and everything that surrounds you, you take your power back, and this book is all about that—giving you your power back. Doing the work and living a healthier, whole, and more fulfilling life is the only power to desire, as it is yours to live within. It is all we truly have and own: our bodies, our minds, our hearts, and our souls.

Living a conscious life is the ultimate way to live. You will regain your health, and you will be able to sustain it as you will learn to understand what your body is telling you, the signs it is giving you, all that it needs, and when it needs it because you will be so connected to it, to everything that it will all become so natural to you. You will arrive at a place where denial will no longer exist in your life, and the magic of your life will be everywhere you are and within you.

The Future of Healing

The future of healing and modern medicine is not new to us; it is instead a return to the ancient wisdom within us that we have contemplated throughout centuries. Throughout my life, I have been fascinated by the writings of some of the most renowned and esteemed philosophers and poets that have ever existed. They, too, knew this thousands of years ago yet contemplated it as we still do today. The written words of our revered past have always made a profound impression on me and my life. It has been thousands of years, and it has genuinely been written for us, time and again, but we continue to miss it. If we learn from the ancient wisdom of our past and the recent past and continue in a new, fresh, and more profound way, profound healing can and will occur. It does exist for you and me. I have proved it in my own life. The magic is not in medicine but in the connection to our souls and bodies. We were born with this natural healing ability. You were born with it. It is not outside of ourselves in any way, shape, or form. It is not in someone else. It is in you, and it has always been in you.

All that plagues us is the delusion that we, as unconscious beings, know more than our souls know. Our conscious selves. Connecting within, without external forces, is one of the most sacred and mighty things you can do for your heart, mind, soul, and body. I know it can feel formidable sometimes, but once you reach this special place within you, the fear will leave you, and you will be from it. The answers you seek and wish to explore are all there for you in the depths of your soul and your very own being. Profoundly and truthfully. It is there for you to experience its beauty entirely, and it is undeniably accessible to you and only you. It is your very own superpower in vast volumes: light, love, peace, harmony, joy, balance, abundance, and ultimately whole-body health and wellness.

Once you master this, you will have mastery over your life and your surroundings. Things will change for you, and if you fear this change, it is more reason to follow through with it. You can and you will because this is where your soul wants you to be, living within it. Your purpose will become so clear to you that nothing will dissuade you from it.

Connection and Infinite Possibility

If you notice within some of the experiences you have had within your own life and witnessed in the lives of others, you will see where fear held you and them back from connecting to what they truly desire and are in their essence. You will also notice that the individuals who defied all odds, followed their hearts, and surrendered to this energy force within themselves found this place even when everyone told them it was impossible. They also found happiness, purpose, and joy. In connection, EVERYTHING AND ANYTHING IS POSSIBLE. There is nothing that you desire that you cannot have or experience. The right opportunities will come, the right people will enter your life, the right places will reveal themselves to you, and the right experiences will all show up for you. No force will be necessary.

And love—you will experience and find the most profound love story of your life. It will be the natural progression of your life as it begins to unfold. All you have to do is connect to this energy within you, have faith in it, trust it without question, doubt, or fear, and follow its lead. Allow it to guide you and open you up to all the possibilities of your life, as I assure you there are so many.

Connection is the foundation of happiness, joy, and love in its most beautiful form. When you feel it, you will know it, and you will trust it. Release all judgments and disappointments of the past, as they served a much greater purpose in your life than you might have realized, but soon you will. They brought you to this place where genuine and authentic change can occur.

Trust and have faith in the feelings you have always felt to be true for you but were too afraid to follow until now. You felt these feelings deeply for a reason, which is part of your journey, life, and soul's purpose. Connect to this energy force within you, stay connected in its presence, and allow it to lead you through this adventure that we call life as it will safely, peacefully, fearlessly, boundlessly, and limitlessly.

It is never too late to find and follow your soul's purpose in this lifetime. Age is not a factor. Connecting to this energy force within you will restore your youth and liberate your soul. You will feel and become ageless. It truly is a state of being. ***Well Being.***

Once you have done this work, you will realize just how important it will be for you to connect with people in a much deeper way than before. You will find more meaning in your life, and more meaningful conversations will be what you desire and gravitate toward. You will find that experiencing true togetherness in all relationships is so much more than the physical or sexual touch, and it is an intimacy that you will never understand until you have experienced it, and you will.

Your life will become far more enriched, inspiring, compassionate, and passionate than before. You will begin to see life through new eyes and experiences that will fulfill not only your heart and soul but your deepest desires.

It is truly one of the greatest gifts of them all. Surrender.

• • •

Your Connection

Can you recall experiences you have had when darkness was more prevalent than light? When you felt most disconnected from yourself and the world? Can you recall how those experiences made you feel? Can you see the lessons in them now, looking back upon them?

Can you recall your experiences where you allowed your light to guide you? When you felt most connected to yourself and your light? Can you recall how those experiences made you feel? Can you see the lessons in those moments now, looking back upon them?

Can you see the difference between your darkness and your light and their effects on your life?

Can you see your connection to your family, friends, and loved ones clearly? Do these relationships support your journey and your evolution? Can you safely see where you need to release some of these connections or create healthy boundaries within them? Can you identify people in your life as soul family? Can you see how these relationships are different and beneficial to you both? Can you clearly see the lessons that your family and soul family came into your life to teach you?

Can you recall times in your life and relationships, where communication was limited or felt limited due to the form it took? Can you see how being personal, intimate, honest, and present in all communications makes a profound difference in your relationships?

Can you see where you can improve your connection within your community and the environment in which you live?

Are there people or places you are drawn to that you have not experienced or met yet? Can you make plans with the intention of visiting these places and speaking to these people?

Where in your life can you connect more deeply and profoundly?

Connect and **surrender.**

Chapter Fourteen

SURRENDER

Releasing Your Past
to Embrace Your Presence

Beauty is a heart inflamed and a soul enchanted.

— KAHLIL GIBRAN

Surrender to what was, what is, and what will be. Surrender to your presence and live within its completeness.

I used to believe that surrender meant giving up on all that I believed to be true for me. I was never quite ready or willing to give up on anything, especially my hopes, dreams, aspirations, and ambitions. This is where I was most mistaken: in believing that surrendering meant just that, relinquishing hope and admitting defeat in my quest to live out my life in the way that I once perceived it should be. As time revealed, that was nowhere near the truth. Over time, and through some very difficult life lessons, I learned that in surrendering, you are not being guided to give up, nor are you defeated in any way. You are simply opening yourself to the power of the Universe within you and the universal energy in all things surrounding you. It did not mean what I thought, and once I realized this and accepted it as my new reality and truth, everything began to shift and unfold for me in profound and extraordinary ways. Suddenly, and without question, everything began to open up for me in ways that I could not have foreseen or created for myself while I was not in alignment with this energy force within me. It has been a miraculous experience and journey for me ever since.

Surrendering Control

I used to have what I perceived to be "control" over every element of my life because I believed it was the only way to achieve perfection. I believed it was all on me to achieve, accomplish, and overcome. Everything that happened in my life, I had to make happen. I did not pause to think that there was any other way. I certainly did not believe that if I did not do something, someone else would do it for me, because, in my life, that did not happen. I was the protector of all things and all people in my world. I created a fast-paced and meticulous life with little time for anything I truly enjoyed, including my family. I genuinely believed that if I paused, my world would stop. In every way, I avoided doing this inner work that I knew I so desperately needed—the work that has allowed me to live the life I am living now. After all, I never really believed that infinite happiness and joy existed for me. I believed that it existed for other people, just not me. I was so very wrong in this way of thinking, and it did not feel good to have these kinds of thoughts. Still, it took me a very long time to succumb to a new way of thinking, as I fought it at every step. Until I realized that surrendering control over your life is not something we need to fear; it is something all of us need to do. It is the only way to open us up to what is for us in all forms. It is seeing in us the beauty that we wish to see in the world. It is also the most trusted way to live within your dreams and the extraordinary life you know you are here to experience.

Surrendering control to the unknown used to put me in a state of utter panic, followed closely by extreme anxiety. Now it is an exciting new adventure that I get to take part in each day of my life and with each breath. I no longer fear it. I have completely embraced it, because what has come from the unknown since I surrendered control to it has been some of the most joyous days of my life. All I had to do was this inner work and then be brave enough to see it through. It was much simpler than I had ever imagined— but it always is when you are walking in alignment with your soul's purpose. Walking against it is not as much fun, as I have come to learn in some of the most difficult ways, as I am sure you have too.

I have always been strong and willful, but fear had its hold on me for far too long. I am grateful that it no longer does. Everything I ever feared about surrendering the control I believed I had over my life did not happen. My world did not end. It began. It was like the world's weight had been lifted from my body in a deep exhale. I could breathe again. I could see in that moment how I had held my breath for almost a decade, waiting for the next challenge to arrive.

Surrendering to the Great Unknown

Life is never what we hope it will be, and for good reason: what is to be for us is far greater than what we could ever imagine or create for ourselves alone. Walking in oneness with the universal energy force within and surrounding us is where all the magic is. Living in the unknown is not like living in uncertainty. Where there is uncertainty, there is fear. Living in the unknown while living consciously is null and void of all fear, as fear cannot exist within the conscious mind. Living consciously and in a state of surrender is where you will feel the most certain about who you are and the life ahead for you. You will trust in ways you have not trusted before, and I know that sounds so cliché, but it is so true. I am speaking as someone who has had some serious trust issues, and for good reason—but I am too well aware of who I am, my surroundings, and my soul's purpose to be untrusting now. I also know and trust that I will not be guided toward the same types of individuals or circumstances as before, because I have done this work. I no longer need to go through those experiences; I have had them and awakened from them and will not allow myself to fall prey to them again.

Trusting in the Universe and surrendering to its beauty means having faith in the bigger picture of your life that you have always known and felt exists for you on some level of your consciousness. By surrendering, you are allowing it to unfold for you, knowing that an ancient wisdom and energy force is at hand and is guiding you through. It will require you to let go of your need to control everything in your life, to accept what is and accept its guidance graciously and without hesitation. It will require you to embrace the present moment fearlessly, experiencing each moment with grace, gratitude, and mindfulness while releasing the past and any concerns about the future. You will find peace in being fully present—to put it another way, you will find peace in *presence*—and life's challenges and difficulties will become easier to navigate. Everything about your life will undergo a significant transformation that will shift you into your beautiful new life where everything is possible and waiting for you.

Surrendering to the unknown, your inner self, and living consciously is the gateway to the evolution of all things, including your healing. You will be astonished at just *how* healing this surrender will be for you and your body. As you tap into this magical and sacred place within you, your energy will return in ways you have yet to experience. You will connect to this energy force that is so abundant and so limitless, and you will feel it within every ounce of your being. It is that beautiful and that powerful. It will consume you in the most profound ways. Your heart will open, and your intuition will be in full force, guiding you to a life you will love beyond words.

Surrendering to your true self is a gift you give yourself that lights the pathway for you to follow through your life with absolute certainty. You will trust the process with an undeniable faith that you have not experienced before now because you will allow yourself to live within the knowingness of your life, and the opportunities will begin to present themselves to you as you move toward them in your light. Being present and patient are one and the same in this process, as patience is presence. This was another difficult one for me to process, as I was not ever, and I mean not ever, that patient of a person. I was turbocharged, as was my life. I see now how, in the agony of patience *(smiling)*, I was evolving, growing, and preparing for what was to come for me as you are now. I no longer see patience as a weight I must carry but a grace bestowed upon me. Had I not been forced to slow down by illness, trauma, and some of the most difficult challenges of my life, I would not be where I am today, and for that, I am most grateful, and you will be, too.

Surrendering to Your Heart

It takes a valiant heart to do this work, and since your heart is courageous and bold, you can trust it wholeheartedly. You always could. When our hearts are open and aligned, anything is possible. When your heart is present in all places and at all times, it is powerful. When we follow our hearts, we are powerful. It is love, and love is powerful. An aligned and present heart brings us our most beautiful moments of love, joy, peace, harmony, abundance, and bliss, beyond words. Being present and aligned is vital as it overrules the mind and opens all the passageways into the universal energy within you. The heart is where we feel the most pain, but closing it off is detrimental to our health and our lives as we wish to live it. Surrendering to the pain we feel is the only way through it. That is where the healing begins. We cannot run from or suppress it; we must surrender to it to begin healing it. Healing is surrendering to the light within you to release the darkness. There is so much beauty in this healing journey. As you become who you are in your most beautiful form through it, nothing is more beautiful than what you will soon come to see and experience.

Surrendering to Your Truth

When you surrender, you will see how resilient you have become. You will see yourself with fresh new eyes and in a whole new light. You will remove any negative self-talk you may have had in the past, and you will live each day in gratitude for who you are, your life, and the gifts bestowed upon you. You will see that you are more than you ever believed you were or could be. You will wake up each day with a newfound purpose and passion for your pursuit. Your life, as you knew it, will be over, and your new life will begin to bring you infinite wisdom and endless happiness. That is what living consciously will do for you. Everything changes most beautifully and most profoundly.

These profound changes will come naturally to you in living a conscious life and surrendering to the events unfolding before you.

You will take action every step of the way. Only, your efforts will be in complete faith. You will not question your actions because you will trust them. You will release all attachments to your desired outcome as you will come to know, with absolute certainty, that you will reach your desired result in a way that will exceed your expectations, the many gifts to you from the Universe. The Universe will support and guide you in living consciously within your inner light and connection to your energy force. Your life force. Bringing your truth into your reality is something that you must do, but you will not be alone. You will be aligned with this energy and living within its light, which will light the way for you. You will trust it, and you will believe in it because you will be surrounded by it.

When you align with and surrender to your truth, everything will begin to flow, and you will start to see the synchronicities that will reveal themselves to you. Things from your past that you could not connect until now will take on a whole new meaning. Things will make sense to you in ways that will not surprise you. You will have many "aha" moments. Those beautiful moments will bring warmth to your heart, a smile, and clarity to your soul. And in many cases, much-needed closure. You will begin to understand why you went through what you had and how the experiences have impacted you both powerfully and positively, even when it did not seem or feel like it at the time.

Surrendering to the flow of the Universe involves being open and adaptable to change. The master plan of the Universe for your life will look different from the one you may have created for yourself, and that is a beautiful thing as it will bring you the most joy, health, and happiness in this lifetime. I once had a plan for my life, and I am so grateful that the Universe showed me a different plan. The Universe's plan was far greater for me than anything I had chosen or could have imagined for myself. We tend to be limiting in how we view ourselves and our lives. The Universe does not see us in a limiting light; until we surrender, we do not realize how limitless we are.

Adapting to this new mindset will come naturally because you will physically see and feel the difference in your body and your life. You have been resilient, you have been strong, and you have navigated your way through it. You have adapted to all the experiences that have brought you to this place, and now you can open yourself up to this new chapter of your life, as it will be your masterpiece. Embracing this transformation and way of life will allow you to become open to the events that will now take place in your life, allowing you to embrace them and accept them without self-sabotaging them. Self-sabotage will be a thing of the past and will play no part in your future. You will not do it, nor will you wish to, as you will soon overcome all the negative self-talk. It will not exist in your mindset because your soul will not allow it—another beautiful element of living consciously and in alignment.

Surrender to Each Moment of Your Life

By surrendering, you will live within the presence of your life. I used to believe that this was an impossible task and that my mind was incapable of it. It took time and patience, but I did achieve this. It took a conscious dedication. As I was working on my mindset and analyzing and observing my thoughts, I realized how useless these negative thought patterns were and how being at war within yourself is silly. As good as I thought I was at time management, this proved that this was time wasted. Something that I loathed. I accepted it for what it was and released it because I knew I would not take it into the future with me. I surrendered to that time-consuming trait and abolished it *(smiling)*. If a negative thought creeps into my consciousness, I rescind it in that moment and the form in which it crept in. If you ponder this, you will understand how precious you are and how this inflicts pain unnecessarily and without merit. It denounces your very being. Your energy force. The ancient wisdom within you. It only brings you unhappiness and feelings of loneliness and hopelessness. Nothing good can come from it, so letting it go was my deliverance. It is the one thing that we all do that we can safely let go of. In surrender, it is effortless because you are in the present moment, not the past or future, where these thoughts originate from.

Surrender Transcends Fear

One of the most monumental elements of surrender is releasing all fear. It will not exist for you once you reach this state of consciousness. You will be astonished at how quickly it will disappear from your life. You will be in a blissful state of shock when it does *(smiling)*. It may take some adjusting to as it may feel foreign to you initially. It took me some time to embrace, as I was sure it would not last; I was sure something would happen to burst this spectacular bubble I found myself in, but indeed it did not. There were moments when I felt fear coming on, but I soon realized I was manufacturing it out of habit and not from what was happening in my life—another "aha" moment. We manufacture our fear by not living in the presence of our lives, not living consciously, and not being in connection with our inner light. When living consciously, we do not manufacture fear or the situations that cause us to feel fear. We know to avoid it when present and open to our inner light and guidance. It sounds unimaginable to live a life where fear does not exist, but we can. You can. Fear is manufactured in the unconscious mind as the conscious mind sees fear as an opportunity for growth and evolution. In this sense, fear has transcended into what it truly is—an obstacle to be overcome and not repeated. Lessons learned.

This dance that we do and have done, with fear, will finally come to an end. You will take your final bow with it and graciously and intentionally move into the dance of your life that will twirl you into the magic that is your life. An energy force without fear is boundless, as you will come to see and feel.

Your unconscious mind will hold you captive until you surrender to your consciousness and begin to live consciously. It is the only way to surrender and eliminate fear from your life forever. You can do this. I know you can.

Healing will happen within the transformational elements of this work. You will no longer be fighting your body, attacking your body, and working against it. You will be in oneness with your infinite self. Your light within. You are healing from your toes to your crown. You will not merely exist within the body you once lived in; you will be whole. All the shattered pieces will unite in connection, releasing the emptiness that once consumed your body. Resist resistance and allow yourself this gift. It is yours. It has always been yours. The life lessons that brought you to this place were gifts, too. You came here to do something magnificent that only you can do. Why resist any of it at this stage in your life? Living as you have has not brought you the joy or the happiness you desire, but you can still have it and much more. Have faith in the Universe and your place within it.

Surrender with Love

You are surrendering in love. If you are reading this book, I know that your ability to feel love and to love others is much deeper and far greater than most. It is why you seek the truth and have the desire to understand it, especially the truth within your heart and soul. Being in a state of consciousness and complete surrender will reveal to you the love that is here for you in all areas of your life. You will see the love you put into this world reciprocated because you will begin to surround yourself with it in ways that perhaps you did not before. You will have a much deeper appreciation and understanding of who you are and what you truly desire in relationships of all kinds, especially relationships where you share your most vulnerable self. Being vulnerable in a relationship is sharing yourself intimately. It is the ultimate sign of self-love and surrender. It is a sign of great strength. Strength in who you are and your ability to communicate who you are to those you love in your life. It offers you and them a safe and sacred place to share without judgment.

In complete surrender, you will know whom you can share yourself with in this way. You will also release resistance to the individuals and relationships you know no longer support you on your journey. It is a sign of self-love and self-protection that will remove you from all that binds you to your past so you can become fully present and in love in a way that inspires you and those around you.

Love, in all its forms, is meant to inspire us. It supports us in our growth, as when we evolve, so does everyone around us. It can also allow the right individual to come into your life to share in life's journey with you soulfully and beautifully.

If you are in a one-sided relationship, you will understand why you engaged in it and you will have the strength to disengage from it now. You will appreciate, without hesitation, that it served its purpose in your enlightenment, and you will surrender to the lessons it taught you. Seeing all painful situations or events in your life as catalysts for your evolution allows you to surrender much deeper. It also releases the pain and the trauma from your mind, heart, soul, and body. It is ultimately where healing of all kinds takes place, in surrender.

Patience

This one word was once so challenging for me to hear and to process. I only understood its true meaning once I reached this place of surrender. Surrender taught me that being present is being patient. When you are living consciously, and in the presence of your life rather than the past or the future, you are living with patience and grace naturally. There are no expectations, only complete faith and trust in the universal energy you are now in. When you allow the Universe to guide you, you will see how everything will fall into place in divine timing.

Surrender will also release you from lifelong regrets because you will realize how valuable those things you regretted are to you now. They were catalysts for change. It is truly the state of being where everything in your life comes together and makes complete sense. Soul sense.

Some people may not be ready to embrace you on this journey but will support you because they know they are on the same journey. In time they will join you.

Surrender is powerfully healing.

We are all here to be of service to ourselves, our families, and those whose lives we come to touch. Surrender and serve with kindness and grace, especially when it comes to yourself, throughout this journey. You have reached the place in your journey where all is possible now. Healing is happening. Be gentle with yourself as you graciously move throughout each day in gratitude. You have come so far, and the miracles and the magic are coming.

The Universe reawakened you
so that you can reawaken others.

Radically accept the power of the Universe within you, your energy force. It is endless, boundless, and limitless. Trust this process. Trust your inner self and guidance. Live consciously within the flow of your life. Resist resisting what you know and feel in your heart and soul to be true for you. Release all fear of the unknown and take each step confidently, knowing you are protected and will have all you need to see this through. The Universe will guide and provide for you; if you notice, it already has. Embrace it. You are here because you have something beautiful to offer this world, and the world needs your beauty and your gifts. Dive deep within your soul to find, understand, and follow through with your soul's purpose in this lifetime, as I know it is beautiful, empowering, and transformative. No one else can bring it to life like you can. We all have a gift within us, and it is up to us to surrender and allow the Universe to work through us and, in partnership with us, bring these gifts into our world when the world needs them most. If you could not do this, you would not have this unrelenting desire within you to do this. A longing that has yet to leave your body and that will not leave your body until you are in alignment with it and bringing it into life and existence. It is your life to live. You have already tried living it unconsciously. Now see what living consciously will bring you. You will be grateful that you did.

When you have done this work and reached the surrender part of your journey, you will find that you are not only ready but already at peace with your past, embracing the present, and excited for the future, whatever it may be. There will be significant shifts in your life, and everything will begin falling into place in a way that you could not have planned for. Divine timing will take on an entirely new meaning. You will feel at home in your own body and life and ready to move mountains in the way only you can.

Surrender and trust
the universal energy within you
because it is YOU!

Beautiful, brave, and bold.

Your Surrender

Can you look at your life and surrender the control you believe you have over your life? Can you find peace in this release and surrender?

Can you release the fear of the unknown and have faith in the light you carry to guide your way forward?

Can you surrender to the desires of your heart and allow your light to guide you forward?

Can you surrender to the truth that you already know deep within you?

Can you surrender to each moment in your life without fear?

Can you surrender to and release the fear you feel now?

Can you surrender in love and patience in all things, especially you and your journey?

Can you surrender and embrace your awakening or reawakening?

*Can you surrender to the power of your **body**?*

part v

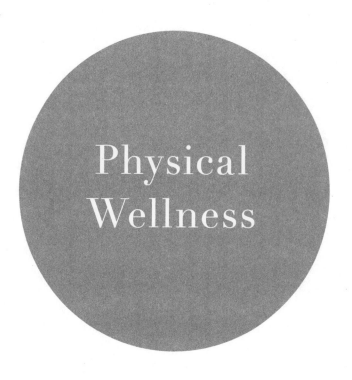

Physical
Wellness

Chapter Fifteen

POWERING YOUR BODY

Emotional Eating and Your Relationship with Food

The point of power is always in the present moment.

— LOUISE HAY

During moments of sorrow and unrest, we tend to gravitate toward things that bring us comfort versus things that benefit our overall health and mental and emotional well-being. Deep emotions bring these moments on, and they can indirectly and directly affect the foods we consume as we tend to gravitate more toward comfort foods rather than nutrient-dense foods. These foods fill a void when we consume them and bring on a plethora of emotions after we consume them, such as guilt, shame, and uneasiness, that are uncomfortable to sit with beyond the comfort the food initially offered.

We have all dealt with this at some point in our lives and perhaps still do occasionally. I have experienced this and witnessed it with hundreds of clients who came through my doors daily. Sometimes we are aware of it; sometimes we are not. As you move through this body of work and your emotions, this will be revealed and healed as it all works together in wholeness.

Emotional Eating and Comfort Foods

Comfort foods are like comfort zones; they do not bring long-term comfort. Living within these powerful emotions versus dealing with them ultimately takes its toll on your body like everything else. If intense emotions are left stagnant, they will adversely affect your body. Emotional eating is one way that they do this, and this is one of the main reasons why you may gain weight and become more symptomatic: because you are not eating to heal your body; you are eating to avoid your body, your mind, and especially your emotions. People eat emotionally even when they are not hungry, sometimes out of boredom, making it more challenging for their bodies to support them in the changes that they seek.

As you begin doing this work and working through your emotions, anxieties, stressors, triggers, and trauma, you will begin to look at food differently, which is why this work is so important. Your relationship with food will change. You will become more conscious of how you empower your body with the food that you choose and consume. You will also become more conscious of your eating habits—the when, why, and how you consume food.

It will no longer be about comfort, boredom, or denial but about eating mindfully and consciously. As you become more emotionally balanced, centered, and clear, your body will tell you what it needs, and you will begin listening to it because, at that point, you will be able to hear it and feel it, and you will not wish to deny it any longer. Your body will start to give you signals as to what it truly needs. You will begin to crave foods that will nourish your body, heal your body, and offer you endless energy—making turning back impossible. This is not to say you cannot enjoy certain foods you love, because you can and will. They will just be consumed from a place of enjoyment rather than distress. See the beauty in that (smiling).

When you become more conscious of your eating habits, you will understand how food affects you and your body. You will be more aware of how certain foods make you feel after you consume them. If a food brings you discomfort, bloating, gaseousness, acid reflux, or anything that feels uncomfortable, that is your body's way of telling you that it is not a food that your body needs at that time. It is not to say you cannot reintroduce it at a later time, but for now, it is not a food choice your body needs to thrive. Your body will guide you in this way if you allow it to.

When I was in my darkest moments, after the heartbreak and my father's passing, I was functioning from a place of complete and utter emotional exhaustion. I was working 24/7 while trying not to deal with all these intense emotions and the sale of my business that consumed me for over a decade. It was a lot to process and let go of simultaneously. I was completely in denial and void of all the emotions of the heartbreak and grief that I was feeling and consumed by. I was running from these emotions and not caring for myself as I was accustomed to. I was living in the void of my life once again. It wasn't until later that I noticed and understood my behaviors during that time in my life.

I did my best to manage through this time and made great strides, but I kept hitting a wall—one of my own making, as I could not define where this behavior began. As I began to process it all, I sought support from a dear friend of mine, Irene Pace, who I knew was an expert in this field. During one of our conversations, we realized it was a behavior I had carried with me from childhood that was directly related to my father. I realized that I was implementing this behavior in my life once again after he had passed. I also realized I had been implementing this behavior with my children, only differently. It was quite the epiphany. It left me pondering, leading to an open discussion with my children.

Irene started her career as a registered dietitian, leading teams at medical clinics and running a private practice. During this time, she saw that, for many people, what was holding them back wasn't knowledge but the emotional challenges they had in their relationship with food. Irene built Pace Nutrition around her pioneering methodology, called Greet the Pull, that helps people understand why food is challenging to them. She has used her method to help hundreds of clients, from doctors to entrepreneurs, change not only the way they relate to food, but the way they relate to their bodies and to other people around them. Many of her clients reach significant inflection points in their personal and professional lives through this work.

In the pages ahead, Irene explains more about herself and her three-step method to help you understand emotional eating and your relationship to it. If this is something you would like to dive deeper into, it will guide you through it as it did me.

Greet the Pull

IRENE PACE'S THREE-STEP METHOD

For countless individuals, their relationship with food stands between them and their health goals. Until you understand the underlying factors influencing your eating habits and the scientific principles governing these behaviors, even the most intelligent individuals armed with well-thought-out strategies and the purest intentions often find themselves entangled in food-related challenges. No amount of meal prepping or superfoods will lead to lasting success if your relationship with food is working against you.

Valentina invited me here because the food behaviors that baffle us are the ones I specialize in helping people solve. The solution has to do with something much more powerful than the science of nutrition: it lies in the profound connection between the nervous system and our eating habits and how stress, emotions, and trauma influence our food choices.

The truth is, you're not bad or weak or broken for eating this way. You reach for food because eating dials down the stress response firing inside you. Eating shifts your internal state and calms the nervous system. It's one way we cope with difficulty or withdraw from emotional pain to return to feeling okay.

You were using food as a tool to help shift an emotional state, to help you connect with your family or somebody important, to help you move through difficult things. It was an adaptive tool that was born out of the best part of you. The most brilliant part of you that wants to survive found food as a tool. And yet, you've been told to feel shame and guilt about using it.

Food was a great fix because it can change how you feel immediately. The part of you that wants to survive doesn't think about weight gain next week or next month or if your dress will fit for your cousin's wedding in July. Its job is to help you feel okay in the moment, and food helps with that.

Specific people, places, and situations can turn on a craving or a pull to food. It can be past trauma, feeling alone, overwhelming responsibilities, a challenging work environment, or troubled relationships. It can be the mounting challenges and responsibilities of everyday life.

The good news is that the brilliantly adaptive parts of you that found food as a solution are still there and you can turn them in the direction of a new solution that is adapted to your life now. Here's how.

I'm going to invite you to a method called Greet the Pull. Greet the Pull gives you a transformational way to approach the pull you feel to eat. Instead of dreading or hating or feeling shame and guilt about your cravings, they become a tangible entry point to a practice that will upgrade your relationship with food, your body, and your life.

When I say "pull to food," what comes up for you? Can you imagine that pull? Can you notice it somewhere in your body? You may even be getting hungry as you read this. That's the pull.

When you find yourself cruising the cupboards, that's the pull. When you notice you're thinking about what to eat, or about the leftovers in the fridge, or popcorn at the movies, or turkey at Thanksgiving, that's the pull. When you drive past the coffee shop and are suddenly turning in, that's the pull. When you're sick and want soup, or sad and want ice cream, or bored and want nachos, that's the pull. Anytime you think about or engage with food, that's the pull. And that's the invitation to all the transformational work that happens from here.

Note some people find they have a push away from food more than they feel the pull toward it. You can think of this as a pull away from food or as a push. Try both and see what works best for you.

It will feel different than anything you've done before because we're not going to start with a meal plan, food rules, or clean eating. We're going to start with gathering a lot of data. As you think about this work, I invite you to think about working in two modes: DiscoveryMode and MasteryMode.

MasteryMode often includes some discovery as well, but in DiscoveryMode, the only thing we're mastering is getting better at discovery. Our goal is to intentionally not change anything yet. At first, we want to observe without disturbing others. Gather data on your relationship with food in the wild. Untamed. Uninhibited. We want to watch it. See what comes up. See what connections we can find to people, places, other areas of your life, your history. Think of yourself as the National Geographic researcher with enormous binoculars tucked away in bushes.

The Greet the Pull method is based on a simple three-step practice, which serves as the foundation for all other tools and techniques. Once you've grasped these essential concepts, they become ingrained in your understanding, setting you on a path to rewire the behavioral pathways in your nervous system and build a new relationship with food. Let's begin!

Step 1: Greet the Pull

When you feel the urge to eat, acknowledge it by saying, "Hello, Pull! I see you, old friend," like you would when someone knocks on your door. You don't have to like the feeling or be thrilled to see it, but simply open the door and acknowledge its presence. This act of greeting boosts your awareness, and awareness is the first step toward making a change.

Let's take a moment to explore why we "greet" instead of "name" or "note" in this practice. When you note or name something, it often leaves space for judgment and criticism to sneak in. You might think, "Oh no, that annoying pull again! I just ate! What's wrong with me? I shouldn't be hungry now!"

On the other hand, "greeting" the pull brings a different vibe. It leaves less room for judgment and criticism and more space for connection, curiosity, and compassion. Noting or naming can feel a bit like a business transaction, while greeting is more like building a relationship. When it's relational, it becomes more approachable and safer, and it feels easier.

Step 2: Get Curious

This step is about creating space and setting the stage for discovery. When you get curious, imagine you've just created a cozy little curiosity container for yourself to play around in, ask some questions, and gather some information about your thoughts, feelings, behaviors, and beliefs about food.

You can go as deep as you want or as surface as you want to at that moment. You get to decide. If you're in the middle of your day and you're doing other things, and the pull to food comes up, you can Greet the Pull and run the practice quickly.

The next time you're greeting the pull, you may have the time and capacity to go deeper. You spend a little more time in the curiosity container and ask more questions and gather some more data.

The full Greet the Pull method includes a series of questions designed to examine the profound connection between our eating habits and how past and present stress, emotions, food experiences, and trauma influence our food choices.

Here's a question to get you started. This one is aimed at exploring hunger and helping you learn to discern when your pull is really about physiological need for food and when it's about something else:

What type of hunger is this?

Stomach hunger: This is your physiological hunger, when your body is saying, "Feed me! I need energy and nutrition!"

Head hunger: Comes from a thought. When your mind, not your stomach, says it's time to eat. "Hey, it's lunchtime," or "Pizza sounds good because it's game day."

Heart hunger: This is your emotional hunger when your feelings are calling the shots. Maybe you're sad, and your heart says, "I need comfort food." Or you are bored, and a meal gives you something purposeful to do.

A few extra notes about this tool: It can be more than one or even all three types of hunger at once. The type of hunger can shift over the course of a meal—stomach hunger may have you start eating, and heart hunger may have you not stop.

Getting to discern what type of hunger it is usually takes some time. Think about it like you're learning a new language. It will feel fumbly at first; it will feel strange, and you will question if you've got it right. As you practice, it gets easier. You'll figure out which hunger and where they tend to appear in your life. As you recognize these hungers, you can better address what's really going on. For example, dealing with stomach hunger is different from handling sad hunger. If you throw food at sadness, it might help for a little bit, but there are other better-matched responses you can offer yourself for sadness.

Here are a few other questions for when you'd like to dig deeper:

What am I asking food to do for me right now?

What are all the reasons it makes sense that this pull is here now?

What are the messages I took away from childhood about food in this situation?

Stay curious, embrace the messiness, and you'll uncover the secrets of your hunger and the reasons you relate to food the way you do. That's where the magic happens!

Step 3: Give Permission

Believe it or not, I'm not going to ask you to try not to use food. Quite the opposite. You were using food as a tool to help shift an emotional state, to help you connect with your family or friends, to help you move through difficult things. And it was an adaptive tool that was born out of the best part of you. The most brilliant part of you that wants to survive found food as a tool.

And since we are going to call on that same brilliant part of you to find new solutions for you now, it doesn't do us any good to make her wrong. It doesn't do any good to take away the tool you've relied on to help calm and steady yourself as we ask you to stretch yourself to do hard things. You get to keep your food tool while you do the work to build out your toolbox to include other things to calm and regulate yourself. It's like taking your child's favorite stuffy away right before they start the first day at a new school. Not only is it unhelpful, but it's also harsh and unkind.

So, "Give Permission" is truly that—permission to eat or not eat. Both are equal. Have the food. Great. Don't have the food. Great. You are a grown-a$$ adult. You get to choose.

Was that statement frightening? Do images of you falling down a rabbit hole of eating all the things emerge? You're not alone. Trust and confidence in yourself to make better and better choices with less effort over time is where this practice will take you. You will get more attuned to your needs and how best to respond in any given moment. When it feels shaky in the beginning, use this question to guide your choice: What's the kindest, most loving thing I can do for myself right now?

Think of this like your kid is lounging around on the sofa. Sometimes the moment calls for a loving boot in the butt to go out and play. Other times, the moment calls for a comforter and pillow and a loving tuck-in for the day. When you know this kid well and are attuned to what's going on in the moment, you will make the right choice. The same goes for you. As you get more and more attuned to what this pull is calling for, you will know when permission to eat is the right thing for you and when the time is right to challenge in the name of growth.

You can continue the curiosity and observe and greet what comes up in you as you give yourself permission. There's usually some juicy stuff there. It may be hard to give yourself permission. There may be fear that comes up, and that's juicy, valuable stuff too.

Over time, giving permission will guide you to build a robust toolbox of ways to look after yourself. Your body will come to know that having needs is normal and healthy and okay. And your needs matter. You matter. And you are worthy of giving yourself permission to offer kindness and love in a moment of difficulty.

I'm rooting for you.

Your relationship with food can be a significant hurdle in achieving your health goals. To overcome this challenge, you need to understand what's behind your eating habits and the science that governs them. Even if you have a smart plan and the best intentions, your journey can be derailed if your relationship with food isn't supportive.

The good news is that the brilliantly adaptive part of you that found food as a solution is still here. You can redirect that adaptability toward a new solution that aligns with your life today.

Follow the practice, put in the reps. Greet even when you feel like going right to eat. Get curious, even when it feels messy and confusing. Give permission and allow yourself to use the tool you've relied on as you call on your strength to build out new ones.

Greet the pull when you get that urge to eat. It's that feeling you get when you think about food, whether it's stomach hunger or a head or heart craving. It's the nudge that leads you to the kitchen or the drive-through. The pull is your entry point into a transformative practice that will reshape your relationship with food, your body, and your life.

I am incredibly honored to write this piece for Valentina's book because it is an exceptional book that will support you in transforming your whole body's health, your life, and your relationship with food. Her philosophy is transformational and life-changing!

Irene used her Greet the Pull method with me, and it worked. If you would like to see how we got to the bottom of my behavior around food in one conversation, you can read the transcript on my website, www.ValentinaGaylord.com.

I still have my moments, and when I do, I indulge, but now it is from a place of choice, not denial. My body knows what it needs, and it guides me, and I listen to it. I gravitate toward healthy foods, but I will not deny my undeniable love for all things white chocolate and homemade pumpkin pie with my 10 cups of homemade whipped cream when needed *(smiling)*. They have their place in my life and always will, just moderately. Eating healthy will become natural because of how your body will guide you and how you begin to feel. Your energy will be overflowing and abundant, and your body will feel luminous, youthful, vibrant, and radiant once again. You will heal this part of your life, and you will not look back.

Your Emotional Eating and Your Relationship with Food

Step 1: Greet Your Pull

Can you acknowledge your pull to certain foods? Can you list what they are and what pulls you toward them? Next time you have this pull, can you acknowledge it and greet it with acceptance and without judgment and inner criticisms? Can you connect yourself to this pull, and what emotions pulled you to it? Can you become more curious and compassionate with yourself, knowing that you are healing this pattern of behavior?

Step 2: Get Curious

What type of hunger do you feel during your pulls? Stomach hunger, head hunger, or heart hunger?

What emotion are you asking this food to fill that you are not facing?

Does this pull make sense to you in these moments? Are you conscious of it?

Were there any messages that stemmed from your childhood behaviors?

Were you able to relate to this food in an emotional way that you can now heal?

Step 3: Permit Yourself

Can you now permit yourself to have these moments, knowing you are healing on this journey and these behaviors will take on a new meaning in your life?

Chapter Sixteen

SUPPORTING YOUR BODY
From the Inside Out

All that I seek is already within me.

— LOUISE HAY

After reading all that you have so far, you can see just how powerful it is for you to do this inner work and the beautiful results that you will see in all areas of your life because of it, especially when it comes to your body. Your body will respond in many beautiful ways as you transform your life with this body of work.

As we enter our 20s, 30s, 40s, 50s, 60s, and thereafter, our bodies evolve with each chapter. That, alongside all that we hear about these ages, is simply untrue. We become manipulated and deceived by our programming into believing so many things, such as our metabolism slowing down, getting back into shape, or it is impossible to even lose weight after a certain age, during illness, pregnancy, perimenopause, menopause, postmenopause, and so on—all deceptions. We can achieve optimal health at any age. I have seen these myths demolished so often by my clients and myself, so I know you cannot believe what you are told about your body in this way, as it is false. As we age, we tend to carry more hidden emotions such as grief, trauma, loss, heartbreak, and many other intense feelings that become stored in our bodies. We can feel these emotions within us, in our bodies, and within our nervous system, so we are aware of them, but until we are ready to process and heal them, we cannot expect results different from the ones that brought us to this place in the first place. The only thing stopping us is our readiness to heal. Our bodies are more than capable of healing naturally, but they do need our support. Our bodies will send us messages, but we must listen and care for them in ways that will support their healing.

As you incorporate this work into your life, it will become more obvious to you. As you heal, your connection to your body will become stronger. When this happens, the walls you have built will begin to come down, and as you go deeper into this work, your body will begin to show you the results of your efforts in so many beautiful ways. Your skin will begin to glow again; your energy will be unearthed and never-ending, truly, as you will have endless energy. Your body will take on a new form, even better than before. You will feel stronger and more confident in your ability to move forward in your life with all of your heart and soul. A new you will evolve from this work, and your life will take on a whole new meaning. You will be in the flow of your life and not swimming against its natural current.

• • •

Food Is Medicine

The food that we eat is a significant contributor to our overall health. If you fuel your body with processed foods filled with chemicals, GMOs, and antibiotics, your body will become problematic. More so with time. Your liver will become sluggish by digesting these fillers and foods. We are all guilty of this, occasionally or daily, but change is possible and necessary to help your body heal in this way. So nourishing your body with mindful and colorful nutrients will become essential to your journey.

When I began working with Anthony William, I realized my daily food intake was not as healthy as I believed. Working with him taught me how to support my body in its natural state of healing. Our bodies are so beautiful in this way as they are truly capable of healing through anything and restoring themselves to optimal health with our support. Anthony has written an extraordinary book titled *Medical Medium Life-Changing Foods*, which goes into great detail and depth about which foods are best for your body according to your needs and symptoms. It is life-changing, just like its title indicates, and I recommend it if you would like to learn more about how to support your body's healing with food.

My own body began healing, and the symptoms that had created so much havoc in my life started to dissipate, when I learned how best to support it in these ways. When I first began, I eliminated eggs, wheat, gluten, dairy, corn, and canola oil products. I removed all cooking oils except olive oil from our home and added coconut oil and avocado oil. I added fruit—a lot of fruit. Please do not fear fruit, as fruit is healing and an essential part of your healing journey.

My diet is mainly plant-based, but if I now eat some animal proteins, they are always wild-caught or grass-fed and free of all antibiotics, animal by-products, hormones, artificial ingredients, and preservatives. It sounds limiting, but it is not.

Consider this: If all of these chemicals are in your food, they will be in your body, too, and your body cannot efficiently process them. Chemicals are manufactured and not from the earth. For this reason alone, we might be more mindful of them by removing them from our daily nutrition.

Foods that are colorful, natural, and free of all these things benefit your health and healing. The Institute for Integrative Nutrition refers to this as eating the rainbow. Colorful plates, because what is life without color? When it comes to food, variety is essential.

Here are some examples of eating the rainbow and its many benefits.

- **RED:** Cherries, pomegranates, strawberries, cranberries, watermelon, radishes, raspberries, red grapes, tomatoes, and heirloom tomatoes. **BENEFITS:** Cancer-preventive, anti-inflammatory, blood pressure, improved heart, skin, and urinary tract health.

- **ORANGE:** Mangos, oranges, cantaloupe, peaches, sweet potatoes, apricots, carrots, nectarines, persimmons, tangerines, turmeric, butternut squash, bell peppers, and pumpkin. **BENEFITS:** Vision health, antioxidant, digestive support, and skin health.

- **YELLOW:** Bananas, lemons, golden kiwi, bell peppers, winter squash, summer squash, passion fruit, star fruit, papaya, yellow potatoes, avocado, pineapples, and dragon fruit. **BENEFITS:** Vision health, antioxidant, digestive support, and skin health.

- **GREEN:** Asparagus, broccoli, spinach, peas, green apples, green grapes, limes, bell peppers, kiwi, and green pears. **BENEFITS:** Cancer-preventive, antioxidant, improved heart, bone, and mood health.

- **BLUE AND PURPLE:** Wild blueberries, purple asparagus, red cabbage, eggplant, plums, blackberries, and purple grapes. **BENEFITS:** Antibacterial, anti-aging, antioxidant, digestive and immune support, improved brain and skin health.

- **WHITE AND BROWN:** Cauliflower, garlic, ginger, mushrooms, onions, potatoes, parsnip, turnip, brown pears, figs, and dates. **BENEFITS:** Cancer-preventive, cholesterol, hormone balance, immune support, and improved heart health.

- **KEY SPICES:** Garlic, ginger, turmeric, coriander, parsley, cinnamon, cayenne, mint, chives, saffron, rosemary, sage, thyme, basil, oregano, sage, and reishi mushroom. Fresh herbs are always the best for your body and the most flavorful.

Love Is Medicine

Loving your body means loving your imperfections too. This body is the only one you have, so cherishing it throughout your healing journey is essential, as it is home to your mind, heart, soul, and body. Your light. The magic within you. It is the reflection of the world within you, and once you begin to bring this world into oneness, all of your imperfections will begin to fade away, so love them, too. They are just reminders and messengers to you out of love and compassion. Your body has not betrayed you; it has not abandoned you; it has not attacked you, and it has not stopped loving you. Your body speaks to you through pain, symptoms, stress, anxiety, pressure, and tension. If you are not listening to it, it will go to great lengths to get your attention. It has to, as it is your only way back to you, in your most beautiful form. Your center. Your soul's purpose and life force. It will not offer you anything but the truth and unconditional love. Your body is love. When you learn its love language, it will guide you so beautifully, and you can trust that.

Self-love, self-care, and your nervous system are closely related. Your peripheral nervous system (PNS) regulates involuntary physiologic processes like heart rate, blood pressure, respiration, digestion, and sexual exhilaration. It encompasses the autonomic nervous system (ANS) and your somatic nervous system (SNS). The somatic system, or voluntary nervous system, is the part of the peripheral nervous system associated with the voluntary control of the body. Movement and muscles. It is also the messenger between your four senses of smell, sound, taste, and touch in your brain. It also connects your central nervous system to your body, muscles, and skin and is involved in conscious conditioning.

The autonomic nervous system (ANS) consists of nerves that connect your central nervous system to your visceral organs. Your heart, stomach, and intestines. It is the mediator of your unconscious conditioning. It encompasses two divisions: the sympathetic and parasympathetic nervous systems. During a perceived threat, flight-or-fight, your body activates the sympathetic nervous system (SNS).

The parasympathetic nervous system (PNS) restores your body back to a place of rest—a state of calm. Most of us live within our sympathetic nervous system (SNS), so self-care is essential and aligned with this body of work. Healing our mindset, our trauma, our anxiety, our stressors, and our triggers takes us out of our sympathetic nervous system (SNS) and into our parasympathetic nervous systems (PNS), where self-care becomes essential. Centering and calming our minds calm our nervous system, relieving our bodies of all perceived threats and permitting our bodies to relax. In this relaxed state, do something that you love to do for your body. Take a lavender bubble bath with Epsom salt, rest in silence, walk within nature, find a peaceful place, meditate, or do anything that brings your soul peace and happiness. Only you know what that is for you, so trust in that, as it is essential in your healing. Your nervous system is vital, and we do not think about how important it truly is to us until it affects us adversely. It always does when overlooked or prolonged for long periods, sometimes decades. When you start to feel tension in your body, learn to release it immediately. Self-care is a beautiful way to do this. Just give yourself love, time, and space to process the feelings running through your mind and body that do not come from a place of love, peace, and calm and release them through some form of self-care that feels good and safe. Your body will thank you for it.

Strengthening your mindset is a form of self-love and self-care. Protect your mindset while healing your body by aligning your heart and soul. There can be no disconnect and no excuse strong enough to derail or distract you, as you can do this, and you will do this for you. The other side of this is far too beautiful for you not to. You will naturally release people from your life to protect your peace. Releasing the people who do not bring you peace and disrupt your peace. If they are unwilling to evolve with you, you will learn to release them. Release them from your life if they cannot be direct, honest, and truthful with you. If they play mind games, disappear on you, or show any cowardly attitudes toward you, release them. If they disrespect you and your journey, release them. Your self-respect and healing journey need to be protected by you and those you allow close enough to you to make a difference in your life.

People are not perfect, and we all have flaws, but there is a difference between people who genuinely mean well and those who are ill-intentioned. You know who these people are in your life, and it is time to release the ill-intentioned ones from your life. Your life, your soul's purpose, and your future rest on your ability to make the necessary changes that you know, deep within you, need to happen. You have known this for a long time, and now it is time to act. Your peace of mind is worth it, and your health is worth it. You are worth it!

When you become whole and complete, you will attract people of the same mindset to share your completeness with theirs. So surround yourself with loving, inspiring, uplifting, supportive, honest, trustworthy, dedicated, and loyal people who continue to evolve alongside you. It will be such a beautiful, magical, and joyful time in your life where you will be grateful that you made all these tough decisions when you did, and your healing will inspire so many others to do the same. You will see that it does not end with you, it begins with you.

Healing with Intention

Be mindful, be conscious, and most of all, be intentional. You have everything you need within you to see this through, so set your intentions and begin. A great way to start is to write down your intentions and place them somewhere you can visibly see them every morning, every afternoon, and every evening. They must be as present as you are. Keep a journal. Write your story, the beginning, the messy middle, and your beautiful future as it unfolds for you. Writing is healing and releasing it all from your mind and your body sets it free, sets you free to evolve in every way that you need to. Make this commitment to yourself, first and foremost, and no one else. It is all about you. It is your time. If you are not ready at this moment, you soon will be. This step that you have already taken means that you are consciously aware that something much more significant is at work for you and happening within you, and you will soon understand just how meaningful that is to you. If my words mean anything to you, know they are for you. For your healing, your growth, your evolution, and your recovery. You are not alone, and you were never alone. Your soul and soul family is here to help you and guide you. All you have to do is believe and trust the process. *Trust the Universe.*

Trust Your Process

Trusting the process means trusting yourself and your inner guidance. Your intuition. It will guide you to your light, your soul, and your soul's purpose. It is such a beautiful and powerful thing, and it is yours. It has always been yours. Embrace it. Trust it. Allow it to lead you through your transformation because it will. As you take these steps forward, the clarity that will return to your life will open your heart and allow you to feel, listen, and trust it. You will feel, see, and experience its magic by trusting it. Magic that has always been deep within you. You will see your life change right before your eyes, so believe it and trust it when it happens, as it will all be forthcoming. Miracles will surround you and compel you forward fearlessly. These miracles bestowed upon you are not of your making, but created by the Universe just for you. All you have to do is do the work. You are building your castle on the other side of this.

Seeing It Through

You already have the courage within you to see this through. You are holding this book and have already taken your first steps. You are now mastering your life, lifestyle, and health and achieving optimal wellness. You will master this. You have taken the reins and are owning who you once were, who you are in this moment, and who you are becoming. Be grateful for how far you have already come and all you have overcome. Life has presented and will continue to present obstacles on your way through this journey, and as strong as you are and are becoming, they will not interfere in the way that they once had much longer as you will begin to see them so very differently. You will understand they are not there to derail you but to propel you forward. Rewrite the meaning and see beauty in it all. Your heart, soul, mind, and body will be stronger for it!

Training Your Body with Intention

As important as your inner work is, so is how you train your body during healing and illness. At first, you may think you do not have the energy to train your body, but do it anyway *(smiling)*. It will help you in ways only doing this work can, from the inside out. When your body is healing and releasing emotions, stress, and anxieties, the last thing you will want to do is add additional stressors with workouts. So, if you are doing heavy, intense, high-impact activities, avoid them during this time. If you are overreaching in cardio, doing 30 minutes or more, stop at 30 minutes or less. If you love to walk, keep it to one hour at a comfortable pace.

If you prefer group classes, try classical Pilates, which is by far the most beneficial form of movement for your body at all stages in life. I recommend you find a studio offering not generic Pilates, but conventional classical Pilates performed on specialized equipment such as the original Reformer developed by Joseph Pilates, and staffed by classically trained instructors with 500- to 600-hour certifications, with whom you will be in the most trusted hands to ensure your success and safety. Gyrotonics is also incredible for your body during this time. When led by professionally trained coaches, these workouts will ease the stress on your body and give you a beautiful, long, lean look. They will also improve your posture, balance, mobility, and cardiovascular health and strengthen your body in a way that will not harm your body or health. Yoga is beneficial, too, when done with professionally trained instructors.

On days that you train your body, only do one workout per day. On off days, walk or swim. Both walking and swimming are forms of cardio that are easy on your joints and don't cause stress to your body or your immune system, which is most important during healing and recovery. Rest days are also necessary. If your body needs a rest day, give it a rest day or two or more. Listen to your body and it will guide you.

Think intentional movement and healing, and you will heal. Your body will be grateful and will transform with you. I have tested and tried everything, and I have seen and heard it all, and I know this is the only way that truly works for you when healing.

Bloodwork and Scans

Having your bloodwork done by a practitioner you trust is very beneficial. It will give you a good understanding of where your body is at and where it needs more attention. It will also give you a sense of your vital organs, hormones, cholesterol, and vitamin health—a good starting point. Essential vitamins to check for are vitamin D, folate, iron, and vitamin B. Essential hormones require a full thyroid panel, estrogen, progesterone, testosterone, and DHEA. In addition to these tests, a DEXA scan might prove to be beneficial to you as well. A DEXA (dual-energy X-ray absorptiometry) scan is an imaging test that measures bone density and strength. It will tell you if you are at risk of osteoporosis and bone fractures, a form of bone loss that can cause bone breaks as we age. In addition, it will measure your body composition, such as your visceral fat, body fat, and muscle mass. It is the most accurate of all the machines in the marketplace built to give you these measurements accurately. Visceral fat is the belly fat found deep within your abdominal cavity. It surrounds vital organs, including your stomach, liver, and intestines. It is not the same as the subcutaneous fat, which is the fat just below your skin. Visceral fat is quite dangerous to your health. Nutrition and exercise are the best ways to eliminate and prevent the buildup of visceral fat. It is astonishing as I have seen high visceral fat levels in people who look incredibly lean and low visceral fat levels in people who are not lean, so weight is not always a factor.

Knowledge is power when it comes to your inner health and wellness. As you do this work, you will witness your own transformation in the most beautiful and profound ways.

This is one of your many superpowers: the power of health and wellness. A healthy body is yours to embrace, and you have all the tools within you to embrace it.

• • •

Your Body

*Can you see where in your nutrition you could make some changes
and additions to support your mind, transformation, and healing?*

*Can you make time for more self-care and self-love in your life?
Can you make a list of things that you love to do that
you feel you and your body will love?*

*Can you implement intentional movement into your
life that you love or intend to try something new?*

Can you learn to trust this process and your body?

Chapter Seventeen

RESTORING YOUR BODY

Rest

Sleep is the best meditation.

— DALAI LAMA

Rest. It is so rejuvenating and restorative and yet so complicated. Something you would not think to be as challenging as it is.

Rest is now predominant in my life. After decades of finding it difficult to fall asleep, stay asleep, or sleep peacefully through the night, I have found peace and rejuvenation in an entire night's rest. But at one time it felt totally foreign to me. Sleep, which should have seemed simple, had become so enigmatic and ambiguous that I felt I would never understand its impact on my life or why I could not achieve it for myself. My lack of rest was overwhelming and at times debilitating, as I knew it also contributed to my many health issues. It made me feel so much worse, and my symptoms were amplified because of it, as if they were not difficult enough to manage already.

Through the years, I tried many different things to help me fall asleep with little to no avail. As my body began to heal, and so did my symptoms, sleep was still my greatest challenge. When I finally healed my body from my autoimmune illnesses, sleep still escaped me. I had read several books on sleep, listened to many lectures, and even visited a sleep specialist. All these things were beneficial in many ways, but something was still missing. As physically exhausted as I would feel from not sleeping for days, I still could not quiet my mind, calm my body and nervous system, and find peace within, no matter how hard I tried. That inner feeling buried deep within me was still gnawing at me. Until I began to listen to it, I did not find a single night of restful sleep. I did not realize it then, but the body of work I am sharing with you here would eventually heal this part of my life as well.

During this time, perhaps surprisingly, I often found I had endless energy. Like more energy than I knew what to do with, energy that I never thought I would have back in my life. Sometimes, I would go three to four weeks without sleep, fall asleep for 12 hours, and wake up feeling like I could take another three to four weeks without sleep. It was one of the many gifts of healing my body.

Sleep, or lack thereof, did not seem to slow me down, but I could always feel it would catch up to me one day. I tried hormone replacement therapy, which I thought would balance me out and allow me to sleep solidly through the night. I tried many different variations of estrogen, testosterone, and progesterone over 12 months, hoping that it would help me balance this aspect of my life and allow me the honor of sleeping throughout the night. It did not. It was a roller-coaster ride of challenging emotions to manage and tolerate. All it did was put 15 to 20 pounds of water weight on me. It not only set me back in my weight, but it brought on feelings of depression, anxiety, and a whole slew of symptoms that I had worked so hard to reverse.

Eventually I withdrew from HRT, as it was sapping me of the endless energy I was reveling in. As much as I desired sleep, energy was my life force and something I could not live without. I then restored my health, energy, and weight to normal by following Anthony William's advice and doing a cleanse he describes in his book *Medical Medium Liver Rescue*. To this day, I consider this cleanse my saving grace. It is my go-to whenever I need to restore my immune system from challenges I have faced since my first recovery, and it has not let me down.

As I began to do—or, shall I say, was forced into *(smiling)* doing—my inner work, I noticed things shifting for me in so many beautiful and wondrous ways, and this was one of those ways. When I finally sold my business and began following that captivating inner light that had been relentlessly gnawing at me for decades, my body, my nervous system, and my life began taking shape. Peace became my new state of mind and new state of being. And yes, I slept through the night for 10 days straight without interruption upon walking away from my studios for the last time. It was so refreshing and invigorating. I had realized that my inner dialogue was what had been keeping me in this constant state of illness, anxiety, stress, and depression, and it was the sole reason why I was never able to quiet my mind long enough to sleep throughout the night or live a more fulfilling life. It all began to unfold right before my eyes at last.

Sleep was yet another way my body tried to get my attention. It shows you just how stubborn I truly was. I defied my body and soul as if I knew better than the ancient wisdom of the Universe! It is our inner knowingness that truly knows it all. I was missing oneness—the key and missing link to my sleep deprivation.

Once I realized this, I began supporting my sleep in new and helpful ways to help me manage as I was evolving with my inner world, as I knew that it would be a process and would not happen overnight *(smiling)*. It would take time for me to work through all that I had to work through, so I had to give myself grace, permission, and the ability to trust all that was happening. Knowing this helped relieve the stress and anxiety of it all. Restless sleep, insomnia, and all that comes with sleep deprivation can be so disheartening and debilitating, but you can and will overcome it as I did.

Of the many things I have tried over the years for sleep support, I will share with you what has worked wonders in my life.

Setting a Sleep Schedule

First, I set a sleep schedule. Through my work with Anthony William's teaching, I had learned his philosophy regarding sleep, and I was always fascinated by how he described the most crucial time for the body to rest and restore. He refers to it as the "sacred sleep window," between 10 P.M. and 2 A.M., and says that this is the most critical time for your body, the time when it does most of its healing.

Reflecting upon Anthony's sacred sleep window, I started there. I prioritized sleeping—or, if I could not sleep, resting my body and mind—between the hourse of 10 P.M. and 2 A.M. No negotiations. No distractions. I made sure that I turned off all electronics (including my mobile) and all lights and set my home's air conditioning to a cool 68 degrees one hour before I planned to sleep. It is much easier for you to sleep when your body temperature is cool, rather than warm or hot. You want to ensure that you are comfortable and have no distractions other than the ones in your mind, which will dissipate as you do this work.

Setting the Mood

Our bodies have a 24-hour cycle, called the circadian rhythm, that responds to light and darkness. When there is light, our body responds by being awake; when it is dark, it responds by falling asleep. Avoiding bright lights or sunlight for at least two hours before falling asleep is helpful, and darkness while sleeping is essential.

This was something I had not considered. Complete darkness was difficult for me initially because I was deathly afraid of the dark. I always have been. I always had lights on, the television on, or something to brighten up our bedroom. Realizing that dark is so important to a restful night's sleep, I bought an eye mask to create the illusion of darkness. Knowing I still had night lights on in my bedroom and throughout my home brought me great comfort in combating my fear until I worked through it, which I did *(smiling).* If you can sleep in complete darkness, that is always the absolute best option. Waking up to natural light is wonderful as it lets your body know it is time to wake up. To enhance this benefit, take a walk outside upon waking or have your morning beverage someplace where you can enjoy some natural light.

The mood you are in before you fall asleep is so important, too. If you are agitated, upset, or anxious, falling asleep and staying asleep will be challenging. Finding ways to calm your mind and find peace before you fall asleep so you can sleep soundly is powerfully supportive. Write, journal, meditate, stretch, take a bubble bath with lavender oil and Epsom salts, and release your concerns, irritabilities, or agitations before lying down. Surrender. I know this may sound challenging now, but it will get so much easier as you begin to do this work as you will feel less and less of these things as you do, and then one day, you will feel none of these emotions as you will be on your soul's path following your soul's purpose. They will cease to exist and no longer affect you in the same way as before. Sleep will become effortless and very natural for you. Not to mention, what once concerned you will no longer hinder you. One of the many benefits of doing this work is seeing things for what they truly are—a manifestation of all you once feared.

Your bedroom plays a huge role in your sleep. Make it work for you. I am a minimalist, so less is more. If your bedroom is cluttered, declutter it. Believe it or not, your space should speak to your soul. It should be peaceful, calm, and pleasing to your eye. What makes you feel peaceful makes you sleep peacefully. Appeal to your senses of visual, sound, touch, and smell. All these senses, including taste, are monumental in our daily lives, though I would not recommend eating before bed *(smiling)*.

For me this was a constant because I drank so much water and tea during the day, at least 80 to 100 ounces. Once I was up, I was up, and falling back to sleep was next to impossible. So I made a few adjustments here, too. I rearranged my schedule to start my daily water consumption first thing upon rising, with warm water with lemon, and to stop drinking any liquids after 6 P.M. I also eliminated all caffeinated beverages at least 10 hours before I planned to sleep. It worked wonders, as I was no longer feeling the effects of caffeine in my system or being woken up in the middle of the night and could sleep through without these interruptions. These small changes make an enormous difference regarding restful and uninterrupted sleep.

Feeling full is yet another way sleep gets disrupted, making it next to impossible to fall asleep. Going to bed on a full stomach, especially an uncomfortably bloated one, will make it very difficult to fall asleep because you are so uncomfortable. It also makes it difficult for your body to do what it does best: heal while you sleep. Your liver will not be at rest; it will work harder than it needs to digest rather than rest, repair, and heal your body. Eating at least three to four hours before bed will ensure that this is not an issue you will face upon sleeping *(smiling)*. If your body is allowed to repair itself as you sleep, this will help restore your body throughout your day.

Supporting the Natural Rhythms of Your Body

Paying attention to these mind-body rhythms—your ultradian rhythms—throughout your day will also help you rest throughout the night. Ultradian rhythms tell your body that it needs a break. Taking mindful breaks throughout your day is very important for your overall health and well-being. If you think about it, you can successfully focus for about 90 minutes, maybe less. After that, your productivity diminishes gradually. Your energy, creativity, focus, and attention decrease. A 15- to 20-minute break every 90 minutes, or more frequently, will benefit your body and mind. It will also refocus and refresh you and your body, making you far more productive and open to your creativity and light. You will no longer overwork yourself or your body to complete exhaustion or burnout because these mindful breaks within your day will revitalize you and help your body heal and stay well.

I had to learn this, as I was always on the go, whether my body was on board with it or not. I was physically present, but drained and mentally exhausted. It is all about healing and supporting your body. It will also help you release stress. It truly is one of the best forms of self-care for your body, and you will know when you need a mindful break within your day.

Some signs that your body needs a mindful break are fatigue, reduced energy, sleepy eyes, foggy brain, extreme hunger, thirst, fidgeting, and feeling annoyed or reactive, to name a few. Supporting your body throughout your day is truly elemental. Rest during these mindful breaks. Go out in nature. Take a walk. Rest in a dark room or put on an eye mask. Breathe, meditate, and find stillness, anything that gives you a break from your mind or the task at hand.

You will return to it more refreshed and exhilarated by giving yourself this time. Your productivity will increase, your body will be grateful, and so will you!

Sleep Duration

A history of less than six hours of sleep a night is linked to insulin resistance, obesity, diabetes, cancer, arthritis, infection, mood disorders, chronic inflammation, cardiovascular disease, and auto-immune disease. It is also related to weight gain and a rise in our cortisol levels. What's more, insufficient sleep drives our hunger. Food becomes fuel to give us the energy we lack, and we can quickly become dependent on stimulants like caffeine, which can disrupt our sleep even more. Seven to nine hours of sleep is the best for your mind, soul, and body. Your body will be able to repair and heal itself, which is one of the many magical and beautiful gifts it gives to us, and all we have to do is support it in the best way we can by making this effort in self-love.

Insomnia and Chronic Hyperarousal

Overcoming insomnia is very important; these things will ensure you do just that. As you release everything you have held on to, this element of your life will disappear. It will no longer be a part of your life or something you stress about. Insomnia contributes to so many things that only work against us and almost always leads to more profound depression, chronic stress, chronic anxiety, and illness. Our goal is to release our lives from all of these things.

Rest Is Not Recreational

Rest is not recreational, and recreation is not rest. Being active during a rest cycle is not resting. Rest means rest. Slow your body and mind down so that you can connect more within and find some inner peace. This will also help you do this work, as you will find more stillness and connection within your inner self and your inner light.

Words are the heart's voice, so say your peace before you rest in whichever way is most meaningful to you.

Your Rest

Can you set a sleep schedule if you have not already?

Have you set your mood for sleep?
If not, can you find ways to do this so that you can rest your mind and your body as you move through this body of work?

Can you identify what you are doing to support your sleep best and what you can improve to ensure better rest? Can you implement some of these ways into your sleep schedule?

Can you make your sleeping environment and arrangements more supportive of your sleep if they are not already? How can you best support yourself in this way?

Are you following the natural rhythms of your body?

Can you make time in your day for mindful, restful breaks?

Can you honor your process into a peaceful night of rest? Letting go of all the thoughts that keep you up at night. It is the natural process of transformation.

Can you speak your truth and make peace with all that keeps you from sleeping?

AFTERWORD

A Love Letter to You

As you journey through your healing and transformation, please know that you are embraced by the Universe within you. You are safe to BE, you are safe to FEEL, and you are safe to HEAL. You are infinitely loved beyond the written words within this book. You are loved as you are in your most beautiful, boundless, and purest form. You are supported in the most beautiful, profound, and ethereal ways as you surrender to this most stunning energy force within your being.

The WELL within your BEING is brilliant, luminous, infinite, and all-knowing. Trust within it as the Universe trusts within you.

The Universe is listening, lighting, guiding, and loving you with every breath that you take, so breathe deeply.

In reverence and love,

Valentina

RESOURCES

As you continue your healing journey, here are some sources of support and inspiration that I hope you may find useful.

Teachers and Practitioners

Randi Marks, Psychic Healer and Spiritual Teacher
www.randimarks.com

Irene Pace, R.D., Food Relationship Specialist
www.irenepace.com

Triona Sheeran, Exploring Soul and Consciousness
www.trionasheeran.com

Anthony William, Medical Medium
www.MedicalMedium.com

Books

Medical Medium Life-Changing Foods and other books in the Medical Medium series by Anthony William

The Menopause Reset and *Fast Like a Girl* by Dr. Mindy Pelz

Supplements

Vimergy, Health From Within
www.Vimergy.com

Pilates

BASI Pilates
Body Arts and Science International
www.basipilates.com

Health Coach Training

IIN, The Institute for Integrative Nutrition
www.integrativenutrition.com

Connect with Valentina

Please visit me online and connect with me on social media:

www.ValentinaGaylord.com

Instagram: @ValentinaGaylordOfficielle

Facebook: @ValentinaGaylordOfficielle

YouTube: @ValentinaGaylordOfficielle

TikTok: @Valentina.Gaylord

X: @VGOfficielle

INDEX

W

Y

ACKNOWLEDGMENTS

Anthony William, Medical Medium, your dedication has guided me through the intricate labyrinth of healing from illnesses once veiled in mystery. I encountered you and your work in my darkest hours, and you illuminated my path, unveiling exquisite and profound truths where answers were once elusive and uncertain. My journey commenced with you and culminated in my healing myself whole. For this, I am forever grateful to you.

Anne Barthel, as my mentor and confidante, you've guided me through the profound journey of bringing this meaningful work to life. Your encouragement and unwavering support have empowered me to explore new depths, and your insights have profoundly resonated with me. Being embraced by the Hay House and Penguin Random House family has been an extraordinary privilege and honor for which I will forever be grateful. Thank you, Anne, Reid, and everyone who has supported and believed in me and the vision of this book.

Steven Harris, you have been an integral part of this journey. Your belief in me and the vision for this book has been an unwavering source of support, and I have admired your straightforward approach to life and business since our initial conversation. I am incredibly grateful to be represented by you.

Elizabeth Hamilton Guarino, I am deeply grateful for your friendship and unwavering support for both me and my family. Your timely outreach came at a pivotal moment when my life underwent significant changes. You have been a guiding light, an earthly angel nudging me toward my true purpose. Your encouragement to share my story and your introduction to Steve have been instrumental in the beautiful unfolding of subsequent events. With all my heart, I thank you.

To my dear friends Jerry and Dian Carmody, I am deeply grateful for your support and friendship. Thank you for everything.

To my beloved family spread across some of the world's most breathtaking landscapes, I extend my heartfelt gratitude for supporting me throughout my journey. Your unwavering belief in me has been the cornerstone on which my foundation rests.

Mitch, I am deeply grateful for your unwavering presence in my world as an exceptional husband, father, and confidante over the past 20 years. Witnessing your steadfast dedication to our family, our children, and your own personal evolution has been a profoundly moving and loving experience. My love and admiration for you are infinite, enduring, and everlasting. Thank you for the beautiful friendship we share, which has endured the tests of time.

Valletta and Luc, my love for you is boundless and eternal. I love you wholeheartedly with every ounce of my being. You became my most cherished blessings from the moment you both entered this world.

To my loving father: your wisdom and your love live on.

To the Universe: to you all is created and sacred. Your brilliance resides within us all. I am forever listening and following your guidance with grace, love, and reverence for all eternity.

Soulfully yours,
Valentina

ABOUT THE AUTHOR

Valentina Gaylord is a CEO, founder, entrepreneur, business owner, holistic health and wellness coach, fitness expert, allergy and asthma ambassador, advocate, mother, and author. Diagnosed in 2012 with the debilitating autoimmune disease Bell's palsy, followed by Hashimoto's disease, Gaylord launched a decade-long personal crusade to not only save herself but to root out an understanding of and a cure for a disease so convoluted and elusive, few answers were known. Seeking out doctors, naturopathic and hormone specialists, nutritionists, and even mediums, Valentina turned her commonly misdiagnosed ailments into a calling that has brought healing, a growing business empire, and a network of prestigious and like-minded colleagues into the fold of growth, wellness, and what she has branded Whole Body Wellness.

Gaylord has dual citizenship and divides her time between America, London, France, and Malta with her family and children with Olympic Gold Medalist Mitch Gaylord. Her love of the arts, music, theater, literature, history, philosophy, music, all things romance, and the Mediterranean Sea has made Europe her home.

Hay House Titles of Related Interest

YOU CAN HEAL YOUR LIFE, the movie,
starring Louise Hay & Friends
(available as an online streaming video)
www.hayhouse.com/louise-movie

THE SHIFT, the movie,
starring Dr. Wayne W. Dyer
(available as an online streaming video)
www.hayhouse.com/the-shift-movie

***

GET QUIET: 7 Simple Paths to the Truth of Who You Are, by Elaine Glass

*MEDICAL MEDIUM: Secrets Behind Chronic and Mystery Illness
and How to Finally Heal,* by Anthony William

*THE MENOPAUSE RESET: Get Rid of Your Symptoms and
Feel Like Your Younger Self Again,* by Dr. Mindy Pelz

*SOVEREIGN: Reclaim Your Freedom, Energy, and Power in a Time
of Distraction, Uncertainty, and Chaos,* by Emma Seppälä

All of the above are available at your local bookstore,
or may be ordered by contacting Hay House (see next page).

***

We hope you enjoyed this Hay House book. If you'd like to receive our online catalog featuring additional information on Hay House books and products, or if you'd like to find out more about the Hay Foundation, please contact:

Hay House LLC, P.O. Box 5100, Carlsbad, CA 92018-5100
(760) 431-7695 or (800) 654-5126
www.hayhouse.com® • www.hayfoundation.org

———

Published in Australia by:
Hay House Australia Publishing Pty Ltd
18/36 Ralph St., Alexandria NSW 2015
Phone: +61 (02) 9669 4299
www.hayhouse.com.au

Published in the United Kingdom by:
Hay House UK Ltd
The Sixth Floor, Watson House,
54 Baker Street, London W1U 7BU
Phone: +44 (0) 203 927 7290
www.hayhouse.co.uk

Published in India by:
Hay House Publishers (India) Pvt Ltd
Muskaan Complex, Plot No. 3,
B-2, Vasant Kunj, New Delhi 110 070
Phone: +91 11 41761620
www.hayhouse.co.in

———

Let Your Soul Grow

Experience life-changing transformation—one video at a time—with guidance from the world's leading experts.

www.healyourlifeplus.com

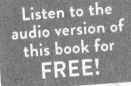